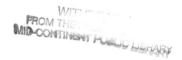

The Climb of My Life

LAURA EVANS

The
Climb
of My Life

A Miraculous
Journey from the
Edge of Death to
the Victory of
a Lifetime

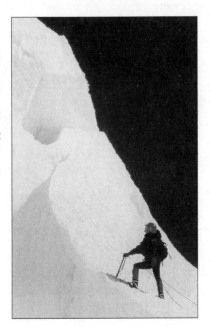

HarperSanFrancisco
An Imprint of HarperCollins*Publishers*

HarperCollins Web Site: http://www.harpercollins.com

HarperCollins®, 🏛®, and HarperSanFrancisco™
are trademarks of HarperCollins Publishers Inc.

FIRST EDITION

Book design by Ralph Fowler. Set in Minion.

Library of Congress Cataloging-in-Publication Data

Evans, Laura.
    The climb of my life : a miraculous journey from the edge of death to the victory of a lifetime / Laura Evans. — 1st ed.
        ISBN 0–06–258658–0 (cloth)
        1. Evans, Laura.   2. Women mountaineers—United States—Biography.
        3. Cancer—Patients—United States—Biography.   I. Title.
        GV199.92.E83A3   1996
        796.5'22'092—dc20   96–9497
        [B]

---

98 99 00 ❖RRDH 10 9 8 7 6 5 4 3 2

I dedicate this book to the Expedition Inspiration team,

to the millions of women worldwide who have struggled with breast cancer,

to the memories of millions more who are not here with us to celebrate this wonderful life,

to all the committed, determined individuals who are working to find a cure,

to the loved ones who have supported and continue to support us through difficult times,

and most especially to my husband, Roger, my family, and my dear friends.

CONTENTS

List of Illustrations ix
Preface xi
Acknowledgments xiii

Chapter 1
   A New Reality, the Diagnosis 1

Chapter 2
   Prelude to Greater Heights 15

Chapter 3
   Transition 31

Chapter 4
   Side Effects 43

Chapter 5
   Rainier Revisited 53

Chapter 6
   Isolation 61

Chapter 7
   Release 73

Chapter 8
   Nepal 83

Chapter 9

Intimacy 97

Chapter 10

Reentry 105

Chapter 11

Kilimanjaro 117

Chapter 12

Building Bridges 131

Chapter 13

Animal Lessons 147

Chapter 14

A Soviet Summit 161

Chapter 15

Expedition Inspiration 177

Chapter 16

The Response 193

Chapter 17

Shakedown Climb 199

Chapter 18

Aconcagua 221

Chapter 19

The Summit 243

Chapter 20

The Descent 253

Chapter 21

Down from the Mountain 261

Epilogue 265

ILLUSTRATIONS

———————■———————

Chapter 1 "Hazards Exist"
Laura skiing on Baldy in Sun Valley, Idaho. Taken one week before her cancer diagnosis. By Nancy Hongola.

Chapter 2 "Injured on Rainier"
Laura on Mount Rainier shortly after ankle injury. By Connie Self.

Chapter 3 "0MTN2HI"
Laura's license plate and motto. By Laura Evans.

Chapter 4 "Bald"
Laura one month after undergoing outpatient chemotherapy. By Roger Evans.

Chapter 5 "Rainier Obstacle"
Laura on return trip to Mount Rainier. By James Kay.

Chapter 6 "In the Hospital"
Laura in the hospital isolation room at Pacific Presbyterian in San Francisco. By Nancy Hongola.

Chapter 7 "In Park After Release"
Laura's victory photo on the day of her release from the hospital, which is behind her. By Roger Evans.

Chapter 8 "Dancing with Children, Nepal"
Laura dancing with Nepalese children on the way to Kangchenjunga. By Sally Chapman.

Chapter 9 "Rog and I in New York"
Laura and her husband, Roger, at a Christmas ball in New York City. The hand-beaded top was designed by Laura.

Chapter 10 "Hiking"
Laura hiking on Proctor Mountain in the Sun Valley area with Baldy in the background. Taken four months after treatment. By Nancy Hongola.

Chapter 11 "Lisa and I on the Summit"
Laura with her sister Lisa on the summit of Mount Kilimanjaro, the highest point in Africa.

Chapter 12 "Rog and I After Treatment"
Laura, and her husband, Roger, three months after treatment.

Chapter 13 "Buster and I Snowshoeing"
Laura and her faithful companion, Buster, snowshoeing in the Sun Valley area. By Bob Ellis.

Chapter 14 "Mount Elbrus"
Laura on the summit of Mount Elbrus, the highest point in Europe. By Mary Anne Regan.

Chapter 15 "The Kick-Ass Ad"
JanSport promotional ad for Expedition Inspiration. Produced by Elgin Syferd/DDB Needham.

Chapter 16 "Kim's Card"
Original watercolor by Kim Howard made into note cards for Expedition Inspiration. Printed by Northwest Printing, Inc.

Chapter 17 "Team at Sturtevant's Ski and Sports"
Expedition Inspiration team at Sturtevant's fund-raiser in Sun Valley. By Willy Cook.

Chapter 18 "Team Photo"
Expedition Inspiration Team below base camp with Aconcagua in the background. By James Kay.

Chapter 19 "On Summit with Radio"
Laura, Nancy Knoble, Claudia Berryman-Shafer, and Peter Whittaker on the summit of Aconcagua, the highest point outside of the Himalayas, radioing down to the support team. By James Kay.

Chapter 20 "Dr. Grant and I"
Laura reunited with her oncologist, Dr. Kathleen Grant, at 16,000 feet. By James Kay.

Chapter 21 "Prayer Flags at Base Camp"
Prayer flags flying at the Plaza Argentinas base camp on Aconcagua. By James Kay.

Chapter 22 "One Step at a Time"
JanSport promotional ad depicting Expedition Inspiration's successful summit. Produced by Elgin Syferd/DDB Needham.

———◼———

Everyone should be passionate about something. Each of us should discover and pursue that one, driving, I-cannot-live-without-it desire. For me it is climbing mountains, both literally and figuratively.

My introduction to mountaineering started on the icy slopes of Mount Rainier and ended abruptly with a serious injury that curtailed any hopes of making the summit. At the time I didn't know if I would want or be able to climb again. But I built back, one step at a time, until I stood on top of the first mountain I was denied.

The empowering strength I derived from being able to figuratively climb back on the horse and achieve my original goal became the underpinnings for the struggles that lay ahead and instilled in me a love and respect for the mountains.

An invitation to be a part of the first American ascent of Kangchenjunga, the third highest mountain in the world, succeeded in hooking me on a sport that up until that point had been only a part-time hobby. Two months in the rarely traveled interior of Nepal and 250 miles over rugged terrain left me with a determination to do more.

However, my life was shattered months later when I was faced with a rapidly advancing breast cancer. After months of intensive treatment, including an experimental bone marrow transplant, I found myself not only struggling to walk again, but also fighting for my life.

The slow process of rebuilding toward a healthy body and peace of mind instilled in me a determination to lead the way for others. The result was the first wellness group in central Idaho and Expedition Inspiration, the unprecedented milestone climb by breast cancer survivors to the summit of Argentina's Aconcagua (22,841 feet), the highest mountain in the world outside of the Himalayas.

This book chronicles my journey from the brink of death and depths of despair to the summits of some of the highest mountains on the far reaches of the planet. It is a story about the parallels between climbing and surviving crisis. It is a manual on following your dreams.

ACKNOWLEDGMENTS

———■———

So often we try to go it alone, but challenges are much easier and ultimately more rewarding with the help and support of others. I thank the many individuals who trusted and believed in me, starting with the handful of close friends who knew even before I did that I could write a book. My sincere gratitude goes to Sally Chapman, Mary Brent Cantarruti, Linda Watanabe McFerrin, and Andrea Gabbard. I also want to thank George Greenfield, my agent; Harper San Francisco, my publisher; and Lisa Bach, my editor, for their interest in the mission of Expedition Inspiration and for their insights, which helped me commit it to paper. For my assistant, Katie Powell, who is always there for me, I have nothing but admiration. And special thanks to Gloria Carras, who set aside numerous evenings to read my book aloud. Mostly I am extremely grateful to my husband, Roger, who spent long and tedious hours reading and editing my endless drafts and who has provided me with a lifetime of support.

I want to recognize all the generous and caring individuals who make up the community where I live, who helped me build back from cancer, and who gave me the strength to pursue my ambitious endeavors. I also owe a debt of gratitude to Peter Whittaker, Paul Delorey, and JanSport, for without their empathy there would have been no Expedition Inspiration. And without

James Kay's splendid photographs and the generous talents of Bill Kurtis and Jeannie Morris, our story would never have been told. Last but not least, I thank all the sponsors and individuals who participated in the success of Expedition Inspiration, especially the breast cancer survivors who made up the very first Expedition Inspiration team, who had the heart and commitment to follow me and my dream: Kim O'Meara Anderson, Claudia Berryman-Shafer, Vicki Boriack, Claudia Crosetti, Eleanor Davis, Patty Duke, Roberta Fama, Sue Anne Foster, Nancy Hudson, Sara Hildebrand, Nancy Johnson, Nancy Knoble, Andrea Martin, Annette Porter, Ashley Sumner-Cox, and Mary Yeo. My sincere apologies to anyone I may have overlooked.

The Climb of My Life

CHAPTER 1

A New Reality, the Diagnosis

Yesterday is already a dream,
and tomorrow is only a vision.

from the Sanskrit

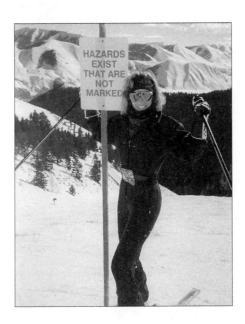

The mountain before me is one I did not choose to climb. I woke up instead at its base, looking up at its towering peaks, anticipating the unknown hardships that lay ahead. If it becomes a contest of wills, I know I can dig deep. I only hope that my husband will be proven right when he says, "Cancer picked on the wrong person."

———————■———————

I hadn't really thought much about cancer, other than knowing that many people die from it. I knew very little about the disease except that it was most certainly awful and deadly. But I had no reason to believe cancer would ever affect me. I was strong, fit, in the prime of my life. Yet in the summer of 1989 breast cancer became a part of my consciousness. At the time, I had no way of knowing that this disease would eventually become the dominant factor in my life, consuming the majority of my waking and sleeping hours.

My new reality started one overcast Wednesday morning in August of 1989 while I was showering at the athletic club after a grueling step class. I discovered what felt like a marble on the front of my breast, a small unexpected lump that stopped my hand cold. I had never felt any lumps previously and had been listening only peripherally to advice about self-exams. This couldn't be what they were talking about, could it? But the lump was clearly there, a lump that hadn't been there before. Or had it? And if so, for how long? That night I thought about death as I lay awake in a cold sweat, more frightened than I had ever been. Was I going to die? I was barely forty. There was no way I could have a life-threatening illness, or so I thought. Funny how invincible we feel, strolling through life, certain that death isn't going to knock on our door for a long, long time.

Much to my relief, my fear was mitigated two days later. I had set up an appointment with the local clinic and went in for my first mammogram. The young doctor on call sent me home smiling. "You're fine. The mammogram showed nothing. Don't worry."

Thank God, oh, thank God, I thought. *I can get on with my life.*

Three months later, however, it was a different story. I was in South Korea on a business trip, working with clothing manufacturers. My trip was cut short, suddenly, by a call from my husband.

"It's Mom. I was at work when Aunt Bert called the house a couple of times. She finally left a message," Roger said between sobs. "Mom had a heart attack. She's dead."

"Oh my God, no." Not Helen. She had been with us less than a month earlier over the Thanksgiving holiday, chipper and chatty as usual. Even at seventy-five, she was flitting around the house tidying things up. How could she be dead?

That night I lay in bed halfway around the world, crying uncontrollably. Roger and I had been together for twenty years. I loved him dearly and loved his mother as I loved my own. *Why did I have to be gone when this happened?* I wanted to know. But Helen's death was not the only thing on my mind. I had felt the lump, another lump, under my arm the day before as I washed the sweat away from my morning run. I didn't want to believe it was there, didn't want to admit it to myself, much less to Roger, especially now.

How will I tell Roger about this second lump? Is he going to lose his wife along with his mother? Am I going to die, too?

In my distress my hand, seemingly of its own volition, moved to the supposedly benign lump in my breast, then to the newly discovered lump under my arm. At the same time, my mind played with the shadows in the room, making them one moment friendly, the next fierce as my eyes brimmed with tears.

The next morning I boarded a flight to Los Angeles, where I met Roger and his brother Steve and my sister-in-law Sandy. The next few days we drowned ourselves in sorrow, sharing bottles of wine with aunts and uncles, cousins and neighbors. I didn't forget about the lumps. Instead, I thought about all my deceased relatives. I was apprehensive that I might see them again sooner rather than later.

I called Dr. Jensen the day I got home, and that Friday afternoon I met with Dr. Campanale, a well-respected surgeon who specialized in breast cancer.

I was perched on Dr. Campanale's high examining table in a white paper robe, staring at a nondescript watercolor painting of a barn in a meadow. The doctor was rolling around the lump under my arm with his fingers, comparing it in size to the one in my breast. I didn't want to look at him, didn't want to see in his eyes the confirmation of my worst fear.

Instead, I glanced down at my watch. My first high-quality watch, a black and gold Concord. For months I had saved money, hundreds of dollars, for this watch, and now it was no longer working, the hands frozen in time. 11:45. At 11:45 my husband and I had walked into the waiting room. We had arrived fifteen minutes early for this appointment, thirty minutes before the nurse had ushered me in here. I stared at the motionless hands on my watch, trying not to read anything into their silence.

I touched the Saint Christopher's medal that hung around my neck. The medal bearing the image of the patron saint of travelers had been a gift from Grandma when I was nineteen years old, heading to Europe for summer study abroad on my first trip overseas. I felt the medallion had always kept me safe. I never took it off until the day, years later, when I sent it to my father. I worshiped my dad, but Saint Christopher hadn't kept him alive, hadn't been able to combat the ravages of an unattended faulty valve in his heart.

I remembered our last conversation before he went into the hospital.

"Dad, are you okay?" I had asked when he finally picked up the phone.

"Yes, Laura, I'm just tired," he responded weakly.

"It took you so long to get to the phone."

"Laura, my heart is slowing down. It's okay. I've had a good life; all of you are grown and settled."

My father died at 3:00 A.M. on May 1, 1987, while I was gently wiping the sweat from his forehead. I had been listening to the rattle in his chest and thinking about the scar that had cut him in half, too late. Dad hadn't wanted the operation. It had been my idea. My inability to let go. Dad wanted to die in bed, at home, but I didn't let him. I convinced him he should have open heart surgery, for us, his kids. When he died I could not release the guilt surrounding the pain and humiliation he had suffered the last two weeks of his life.

After Dad died, I took back Saint Christopher, finding him lovingly hidden in Dad's top drawer under his jockey shorts and linen hankies. As I felt Saint Christopher's outline on the medallion, I wondered if he would be able to help me now.

So much sadness, I thought, as I tried to ignore the doctor's probing hands and the reason I was sitting there. I wondered if the lingering pain of Dad's death had somehow contributed to the lumps, to the disease that no doubt was growing in my body. When Dad died, I felt a huge loss, an emptiness that could not be filled. He had taken so much pride in everything I did. Dad had been my biggest supporter. He gave me strength. I needed that strength now as I sat, rigid, waiting for the exam to end.

Dr. Campanale decided to do a needle biopsy. Isolating the lump in my breast, he carefully stuck a long needle into it and unsuccessfully tried to extract fluids. He withdrew the needle, set it down, and spoke.

"I'm going to schedule a surgical biopsy," I heard Dr. Campanale say. "Just routine, to be on the safe side. I don't think you have anything to worry about."

A biopsy. That's it, then. Maybe it would show nothing. But I knew better. There had been no indecision on the doctor's part. Two lumps. A biopsy. I was in trouble.

I dressed slowly then joined my husband, Roger, in the waiting room. I informed him of the upcoming procedure, set for first thing Monday morning, three days away. Roger held me, not saying a word. We were both in shock. This couldn't be happening. He took my hand, and we walked out of the hospital to the parking lot. We were lost in our own private thoughts, both of us wishing we had been told something more concrete. Was I going to be okay? If not, what could I, could we, expect? It was going to be a long weekend.

I looked at my watch again. Still 11:45. Time standing still.

The next two nights I slept fitfully, but the night before the biopsy, I did not sleep at all. My thoughts were preoccupied with death and life and all the things I still wanted to do. I was terrified of the impending prognosis. What would tomorrow bring? What would I have to endure? What would happen to my marriage and career? Was I really sick? I didn't feel sick.

The same gnawing fears filled my mind that morning as I lay in the hospital. I fought the drugs, struggling to stay awake, frightened of what the doctor might find. To no avail. Later I was told I had been given enough sedatives to knock out a cow. So I lay peacefully, partially reclined, on the paper-covered gray vinyl table on which they do in-office procedures. My face was concealed behind a white sheet, lest I wake too soon, while they cut open my breast.

"Just routine," I had been told. "Not to worry."

But I did worry. As the narcotics took effect, I remembered Grandma, who had died of colon cancer. She had died a slow, agonizing, humiliating death. Mom had found her crawling around the floor of her hospital room, naked and disoriented by drugs, looking for a way out of her pain and misery. I loved Grandma, and I hated to see her life end that way. Would that be my fate? Crawling around on the floor, drugged, dying?

■ ■ ■

When I awakened, I was initially aware only of the smallness of the room. It seemed to have somehow decreased in size, the walls closing in while I slept. With some effort, I willed my eyes open, shifting their focus to my doctors. They were both ashen, as white as the sheet that covered my breasts. In the stillness of that moment, I heard only one word, the one word that hung in the air between us, as if suspended by its own invisible force. *Cancer.* The death word. The doctors were staring at the beaker of solution into which the biopsied lump had been dropped. I was unclear how the solution worked, but it had somehow sealed my fate.

I looked at Dr. Jensen, the one who had sent me home three months earlier, in September. He had been so confident then. He would not look at me now. Instead, his eyes were trained on the glass jar that held the lump that had just been removed from my breast. He looked sick to his stomach—ghost sickness, maybe. He had been wrong, and he knew it. Oh, God. I was instantly totally conscious, searching the faces of each doctor for any sign of hope.

They seemed as confused and disoriented as I was. Cancer. *Color of casket, madam?* I thought morbidly.

"Get dressed, Laura, we will talk in my office," I heard through the haze of my anguish. Minutes later, dressed and seated, dazed, beside my husband, facing a wall of degrees and Dr. Campanale's serious face, I heard the voice again. "Laura, do you understand what I'm saying? A two-centimeter tumor, bigger than we thought, an active garden variety cancer."

Garden variety? Broccoli and carrots came to mind. How could any cancer be considered garden variety? "One out of every eight women. We don't know why. Mammograms miss. Schedule you for surgery . . . oncologist . . . chemotherapy . . . will to live. . . ."

The words registered slowly, as if they were being filtered through another being. This wasn't me sitting here. This wasn't my life he was talking about. It couldn't be. I had always been strong and healthy. *Does anyone survive this disease?*

Surgery was scheduled within a week to remove the malignant tumor, surrounding tissue, and lymph nodes. That night, and most of the following nights, I didn't sleep. On some intellectual level the diagnosis had registered, but I couldn't quite grasp the reality that I had cancer. It seemed impossible that my life would change. Drastically. I was numb. I could recall the fear I had felt three months earlier waiting for the results of my mammogram and the joy I had felt when I was told there was no indication of cancer. It seemed so long ago.

I went through the motions of working, trying to block out any thoughts of the impending operation and what it might reveal. I thought about a mountain climb I had planned and of the friends with whom I would be climbing. I reflected on the mountaineering saying, "Hope for the best and prepare for the worst." I tried very hard to hope for the best, but I was frightened.

On a frigid Monday morning in mid-December, I entered the Moritz Hospital in Sun Valley, Idaho, side by side with my husband. I was barely able to breathe. I had spent the previous half hour showering, scrubbing every inch of my body, perhaps hoping to rid myself of any more, as-yet-undetected, cancer. An hour later, I was wheeled into the operating room.

Even though I was covered in blankets, the impartial and penetrating cold of the metal table on which I lay chilled me to the bone. My stomach knotted as I scanned the machines and surgical implements, sterile and sparkling, ready to go to work. The doctor had already prepped me, "You'll be out for a few hours. I won't know whether I need to do a mastectomy until I get inside and see what is going on. I'll be by to talk to you later." I lay there frozen, unable to respond.

As the anesthesiologist went about his business, my eye caught a cartoon taped to the wall. In characteristic "Far Side" style, it pictured an operation in progress during which some part of the patient's innards go flying across the room. "Better grab that, we may need it later," read the caption. As I drifted off to sleep, I reflected how that would not have been my choice of humor, considering the circumstances.

I woke up two hours later afraid to move. I felt stiff and uncomfortable and uneasy about what was left of me under the sheet. I had always been proud of my body, of my level of fitness, and of the muscle tone I had tried so hard to maintain. And of course, my breasts. I couldn't tell, wasn't even sure I wanted to know, if they were still there. Even more gnawing was the threat that the cancer had spread. What if it was in my lymph system, my bones, my lungs?

I thought about my career in fashion design, all the hard work I had invested. I thought about the endless deadlines and nonstop travel. I thought about the stress of juggling all my clients and the inevitable and frequent problems that arose in manufacturing. Had I pushed myself too hard? I also thought about the satisfaction I derived from the creative process, the many jackets and sweaters and suits that were a result of my handiwork. And I knew none of it mattered any longer. Only one thing was important. My life.

Dr. Campanale arrived shortly after I awakened. He looked down at me and smiled, "Everything went well. I didn't perform a mastectomy, primarily because of your implants," he informed me. "I took all of the breast, however, but your breasts aren't that big. You'll have a dent, which can be filled in later. We'll get the rest of the test results back in four or five days."

I thought about my decision to get implants, three years earlier.

"Rog, I'm going to get breast implants," I had announced to my husband one evening while dining on grilled swordfish and new potatoes.

"You're kidding," he had said in disbelief. "I thought you said you'd never mess with your body."

"I changed my mind," I replied. "I work out all the time so I'll have a nice body, and the one thing I can't do anything about are my breasts. My pecs get bigger, but not my boobs. I'm ready. Why not? I think I would enjoy them. Wouldn't you?" I queried between mouthfuls of food.

It didn't take much convincing. The next day I came home with an armload of girlie magazines, and Roger and I pored over them in bed, giggling like children, picking out my new perfect breasts, the bigger the better, within reason. How irrelevant it seemed now. How insignificant.

It was two weeks before Christmas when I first called my mother, sisters, and brother to tell them I had cancer. Merry Christmas! In many ways, I had been the strongest in the family.

The most likely to live to be a hundred. Now I might not live out the coming year. And what would this mean for my sisters? Would they be next?

Mom was stunned. Her only reply: "Parents are supposed to outlive their children. This isn't fair."

Fair. A friend in southern California who had been through her share of tough breaks had once said to me, "Fair? The fair is in Pomona, October 12th through the 16th." She'd had a good point. What is fair? I understood how tough this would be on Mom and on the whole family.

The battery of tests following surgery came back with nothing but bad news.

"Fast growing . . . estrogen negative . . . metastasis . . . eleven positive lymph nodes . . . 15 percent chance of surviving the next three to five years."

Roger and I discussed my will. Did I, in fact, have one? Was it current? Not something I had spent much time thinking about.

Now all I could think about was the cancer. Why? How did this happen? I thought I was good at stress management, taking time out for myself. I was happy. All past tense. Was I going to die now, so young? My friends had dreaded turning forty. Not me, especially not now. *Lord, can I please see forty-one? Would fifty be too much to ask?* What had I done wrong? When had I slipped up and allowed cancer to take over? What could I, should I, have done to prevent it?

There were, of course, no answers. The only question that remained was, What do I do now? I had no idea. Except that whatever I would end up doing would definitely be different from what I had planned.

I was supposed to be training for a climb up Kilimanjaro with Peter Whittaker, one of the premier mountain-climbing guides and a longtime friend. This was going to be my first major summit. I had become hooked on mountaineering, drawn to the solitude of the sport, the rigorous demands, the discipline. I reveled in the quiet communion with nature, feeling at one with the powerful yet seemingly sedentary beast beneath my feet. On the side of a mountain, looking out at layers of peaks and valleys, which changed in color like chameleons and were interspersed with downy white clouds, I would fill my hardworking lungs with fresh mountain air and feel more at peace than at any other time in my life.

I thought about my very first climb and how it had changed my life forever.

CHAPTER 2

Prelude to Greater Heights

Our strength is often composed of the weakness we're damned if we're going to show.

Mignon McLaughlin

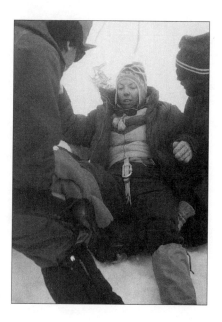

Today is one of those days you never want to forget. Fifty degrees, clear and sunny, with fluffy cumulus clouds scattered among the hilltops. I went for a nice walk, and it gave me a chance to reflect. In the high country I find a solitude, a quiet strength. There is a majesty to mountain ranges. They rest stoically, beautifully serene, while the rest of the world scurries by. One can gain strength in the mountains.

———————■———————

The bus labored up the winding road, slowing down even more on the steeply arched switchbacks. I gazed out the window into dense greenery. My depth of vision was obscured by centuries-old fir trees that could have been Christmas trees if they hadn't gotten skyscraper tall, blocking out the sun and clouds and all indications of the weather.

Around me I could hear the anxious voices of the strangers who would become my teammates, chattering about their level of fitness, how hard they had trained, the challenge that lay ahead. Soon enough I would know these people, albeit briefly. But for now, I insulated myself from their energy, from their concerns, preferring to reflect on why I was here.

I had never thought about mountain climbing, not until Lou Whittaker brought it up. Bigger-than-life Lou, much like the redwoods that now blurred into a field of green out my window. One cannot meet Lou or his twin, Jim, without being taken aback by their sheer brawn. At over six feet four inches, with massive chests and slender waists, the brothers tower over the average person. Raised in the mountains around Seattle, they have as much mountaineering experience as any two people alive. And Lou, especially, likes to share his passion with others. Through Lou's guide service, Rainier Mountaineering, he has led thousands of individuals up Mount Rainier, instilling in each of them (to varying degrees) the inherent benefits of taking risks, confronting fear, and living life to the fullest.

Lou and I both worked as consultants at New Balance, a sneaker company specializing in active footwear and apparel, and there he had talked me into trying mountaineering.

"You ought to come out and climb Mount Rainier, Laura. You'd be good at it," Big Lou had tried to persuade me at a company sales meeting in January of 1983. "You're strong physically and like a challenge. JanSport, the outdoor gear company, has two dealer seminars in late June. You should go on one of those. We would comp your way."

Lou was always trying to talk someone into climbing Rainier. I laughed at his persistence and the prospect of climbing. "I've never climbed before, Lou."

"That doesn't matter. Most of the people who go on these seminars have never climbed before. We teach you everything you need to know," he replied.

I'll bet, I thought. Lou likes women. It seemed to me he was always trying to persuade women to go climbing. Yet the idea piqued my curiosity, and without much more effort, he had convinced me that this was something I should try. So here I was, five months later, on this bus with thirty people I didn't know, heading off on an adventure. *Good stuff,* I thought, *pushing the envelope.*

I grinned as a deer, intent on the grass it had been eating, looked up startled and shot back into the forest, vanishing in seconds. In the city I missed the aura of nature, the wildlife, the small surprises, the soothing embrace. Roger and I had moved from Denver to Boston a year ago, and I still longed for a yard, the mountains, and Clancy, the springer spaniel we had had to leave behind. But Boston was fascinating, packed with history that had never seemed real until I was suddenly living in the middle of it. And we resided in an almost regal brownstone atop Boston's venerable Beacon Hill. We had bought the main floor of an 1850s mansion and had converted it into our home. But we had no yard at all and only a few houseplants that had, remarkably, survived the move. We certainly had no mountains.

The trees flashed by my window as the bus meandered higher and higher. I could feel the air getting cooler. What would this mountain climbing be like? Had I trained hard enough? I had been running daily for at least an hour at a time. I had also sought out all the stairs I could find, making frequent trips up and down them with a thirty-pound pack on my back. Well, ready or not, here I was. I registered the voices around me, allowing their nervous energy to somehow assuage mine.

"I've trained really hard for this. Biking twenty miles a day, longer on the weekends," one of the guys was saying.

"I ran a lot, especially stairs, at least three, four times a week," reported someone else.

"Did you work out with a pack? We have to carry everything to Camp Muir, halfway up the mountain. I hear that's as tough as going to the summit," one of the women added.

"God, I hope we get good weather. This could be miserable if we don't," yet another person observed.

"I'm not sure about this," a young woman in the back timidly offered. I turned to see who was speaking and found myself looking into a pair of dark, apprehensive eyes. They were not unlike the eyes of the doe we had just passed.

"This was my idea," spoke the young man seated next to her as he gave her shoulders a squeeze. "I gave this climb to my wife as an anniversary present," he announced proudly, grinning at her and at all the other faces now pointed in his direction.

"I was hoping for a diamond," she retorted with more than a little sarcasm, looking at no one, preferring the view out the window instead or perhaps wishing she could turn that view into something else.

Rounding the last corner into the parking lot at the Paradise Inn, Mount Rainier unfolded before us in all its jaw-dropping magnitude and splendor. The Native Americans called it Tahoma and refused to climb it, believing that spirits lived up there. I was starting to wonder if the Indians weren't the smart ones.

"It sure is a big fucker," one of the men behind me said quietly.

Once we and our packs were all inside the wooden A-frame building that houses Rainier Mountaineering, Lou began to question us on what gear we were carrying. Months earlier, we had each been mailed a list of all the items required for the climb. Long underwear, tops and bottoms, a fleece or wool layer, down jacket, rain gear, hat, gloves, sleeping bag, crampons, ice ax, water bottles. . . . I had gone over the list so many times I had it memorized. But Lou didn't know that. When he reached me, he stated, "Take everything out, Laura. I want to make sure you have all the items you need."

I looked at him, wishing desperately that I had assembled two packs. Lou, knowing me only as a fashion designer who was always dressed to the nines, no doubt expected that I would have included a makeup mirror, hair dryer, maybe even some pink froufrou slippers shaped like bunnies. I would have loved, just once, not to have taken this so seriously. I could have, should have, loaded up a fake pack full of such things, my real bag stowed somewhere out of sight in the corner.

Our checkout went quickly, and we were soon on our way, forty pounds on our backs, ski poles in hand. The weather gods shined down on us as we made our way through fields of wildflowers and up the massive rock steps that decades earlier had been maneuvered into place, thus protecting the terrain. Two marmots playfully duked it out to our left, enjoying the bright sunny day.

A light stream of water washed over the rocks in Pebble Creek, which we hopped across, from one rock to another, before reaching the Ingraham Glacier on the other side. Now it was snow, forever, an endless uphill stretch of white. Boulder outcroppings added relief to the monotonous terrain, but it became impossible to judge if the next patch of stone was close or far away. All of us hoped that the upcoming rocky ledge would be the perfect spot for a break. I put my head down, refusing to get lured into thoughts of resting, and concentrated instead on rest stepping, locking my back leg, moving only one leg at a time, minimizing my exertion. I focused on my pressure breathing. Fill up the lungs, purse the lips, blow. I matched my breaths to my steps. Fill up the lungs, purse the lips, blow. We would get there when we got there.

Every hour we stopped, gladly disengaging ourselves from our packs, then plopping them onto the snow field to be used as seats. We quickly loaded up on water and gorp or candy, having learned at the first rest break that we would not be here long. "The body cools down and the muscles stiffen up," we had been informed.

There wasn't much time for conversation on our breaks and not much to say. Everyone was trying so hard to stay warm, hydrated, and fed and not show any sign of weakness. We were all aware from Lou's preclimb pep talk that not everyone would make it to the summit, especially if he noticed any of us faltering. Depending on where we were on the mountain, we could be turned back, left in the bunkhouse at Muir, or (God forbid) strapped to the side of the mountain in a sleeping bag. I was determined not to suffer any of those indignities.

Finally, after five or six hours of flat-out endurance, we crested the one remaining hump that welcomed us into base camp at Muir. Whittaker was waiting to greet us.

"You did it!" he smiled broadly when he saw me, giving my sweaty body a bear hug.

I looked around our camp for a spot to drop my pack, relieved to have that leg behind me but also feeling good. *I'm going to make it,* I thought. The rest of the team staggered in and received the same hearty welcome as I had. We shed our packs and got into more comfortable shoes, then nestled into a tilted wall of rocks that was an amphitheater to the rolling hills and mountains stretched below us. As we caught our breaths and rehydrated, we realized that a few stragglers, or at least one climber and a guide, were still toiling up the slope.

While waiting for our final team member, we assessed our new, temporary digs. Base camp was basic. A square makeshift wooden hut would serve as our bunk room. Behind it, perhaps twenty yards away, sat the outhouse, farther away than I would have liked, but then I was sure it didn't smell too wonderful. Probably best where it was. Six feet above us sat the cook shack, a rustic, Himalayan-style stone building the size of a small kitchen. There the guides would prepare our meals, talk about us, and sleep. From our vantage point, we looked straight across at Mount Adams and the flattened top of Mount Saint Helens. I remember seeing the photo that a local photographer took of a fellow climber right here on this mountain. Incredibly, he snapped it just as Mount Saint Helens blew, the eruption knocking her off her feet, even at this distance, sixty miles to the north. Amazing.

We sat resting, taking in the incredible panorama. Before we knew it, an hour had passed, and at last our final team member came into view over the mound of snow in front of us. It was then that I recognized her, the reluctant wife. *I bet she's not too happy at the moment about her big gift,* I reflected. I barely registered that thought when she broke into a tirade.

"Son of a bitch . . . anniversary present . . . asshole . . . divorce . . . awful . . . goddamn you . . . prick . . . divorce . . . "

"I don't think she liked her anniversary present," the guy next to me whispered.

"No kidding. I think a diamond might have been a better call. Don't think he's going to get lucky tonight," I whispered back. Later I heard that they did divorce and that she, not surprisingly, gave up climbing.

We were on a weeklong seminar designed to teach novices like myself "the ropes." Each day we would concentrate on a different mountaineering technique until we had all mastered it or at least come close. We learned how to strap the metal spiked crampons to our boots and to travel, on treacherous slick slopes, roped together. We learned about mountain safety—how to get out of a crevasse and how to help others do the same. I think the guides particularly enjoyed instructing us on how to perform ice ax arrest. If someone should fall as we headed up the steeper slopes to the summit, it was essential that we knew how to stop or arrest that person's descent. To ensure that we could do this from any position, the guides would have us lie on our backs upside down, head first on the side of a vertical slope, while they held our feet.

"Just swing your legs around, plant your ice ax, then kick in your feet," they would say with authority.

Yeah, right. I did not look over the top of my hat at the icy slope that lay on the other side of my head. I had seen it while standing up. That was scary enough. I lay looking straight up at the sky instead, hoping that maybe God was watching and would take mercy. *This wasn't what I expected, really.*

"What if we keep sliding and end up in one of those big gaping crevasses down there?" I inquired, trying to glean some inspiration from the clouds overhead.

"You won't. Just relax," came the response.

Relax?! I wondered what these guys did off-duty.

Each night we would return tired, wet, and exhilarated to the modest, handmade structure where we would eat and sleep. Each person had his or her two-foot-wide space on the wooden shelves that lined one wall. Here we had rolled out sleeping pad and bag and arranged toothbrush, book, diary, snacks, and clothing. I have since heard about Japanese sleeping compartments or drawers, which must have a similar feel.

Dinner consisted of a big pot of noodles or a rice mixture that you would never make at home but that tasted delicious after a long day in the mountains. This was followed by chocolate bars.

Crammed into that small hut, eating mush out of a plastic bowl, we felt a common bond. After all, we were budding mountaineers learning how to keep ourselves and one another alive. But at the heart of it, we were still strangers, and our communications were basic.

"Did anyone else hammer themselves with their ice ax?" asked one of the guys. With thirty of us up here, pretty much dressed alike, it was tough to tell who was who.

"I cut a gash in my rain pants," a voice mentioned from the corner of the room. "Does anyone have one of those repair kits?"

"I wonder what the weather will be like tomorrow. When do you think we will attempt the summit?"

Occasionally someone would tell a joke. Maybe even a good one. And usually Lou would pop in to tell us a good-night story about one or another of his climbing escapades. Sometimes I would read a chapter in a paperback thriller or record the day's events in my diary, but sleep would come quickly.

And so our week went, until the night before the team would attempt the summit. That evening, due to events earlier in the day, I found myself wide awake, not in anticipation but in pain, knowing I would not be one of them.

I sat with my back against the wall, my legs extended straight out in front of me, my boots still on. I remained stock-still, not daring to move, not wanting to jar my shattered and swollen ankle, which lay limply on the wooden shelf that was our bed. I could hear my friend, Amber, snoring lightly next to me and the others, harmonious in the distinctive sounds of sleep.

I thought of Roger, on a boat with his buddies somewhere between southern California and Catalina Island. A little tit for tat—mountain climbing for me, fishing for Rog. I remembered our phone conversation the night before my bus ride up here.

"You be careful," were his closing words.

"I will. No problem," I had replied confidently.

Now I stared at the old wooden door of the hut that led to the snow white glacier and on to the crevasse where we had practiced that afternoon. Over and over I relived every moment of the previous hours.

"Let 'er rip," guide Robert Link had said.

Okeydokey, I had thought.

"Yahoooooo!" I had replied, hurling myself forward. I had felt my body, weightless, flying over the crevasse below, the wind catching the edges of my jacket but not slowing me down. I'd sailed toward the ice wall on the other side, legs extended out in front to stop me.

This had been my first attempt at a Tyrolean traverse, a suspended glide over the vast chasm in the glacier by way of a taut rope to which I and my waist harness were secured with a small metal carabiner.

How exciting! What fun! I thought.

Big Lou's head had whipped around the minute I hit, as the unmistakable sound echoed down the frozen canyon to where he stood, looking up from the floor of the crevasse.

There had been no pain then, just the deafening crack, like a tree felled in the forest, snapped from life. Limply I had bounced off the wall as two of the guides reached to grab me, fearful that my harness might somehow release, plunging me to the icy depths below.

Lou was suddenly there to assist, cradling my body with his mammoth arms and resting me on the snow out of harm's way.

"Does it hurt here?" Lou asked as he gingerly felt the sides of my leg.

"Yes."

"Here?" His hands moved around to the back of my ankle.

"Yes."

"Get some more clothes on her," Lou commanded.

Soon I was layered in down pants and jackets and wrapped in a sleeping bag to avoid any chance of hypothermia. Amazingly, I was calm, perhaps because of the efficiency with which the situation had been handled or perhaps because of shock. I couldn't feel any real pain, not at first, not physically or mentally. As I lay there bundled up on my glacier mattress, with the clouds closing in and a feather-light dusting of snow on my face, I didn't think about anything at all.

"We'll send a couple of guides up for the sled. It won't be long. Try to relax," I heard Lou say. But I already had.

By the time the rescue sled arrived, the intermittent snow-flakes had turned into a full-fledged whiteout. The difficulty of getting the team back to Muir safely, while at the same time haul-ing me out, had increased dramatically. I lay on my back, helpless, as three rope teams of climbers, tied to the litter that supported my body, inched along the steep snowpack. My mind revisited the route coming down from base camp, and I realized, with no small amount of distress, that we had crossed a narrow snow bridge that was merely a temporary causeway between two bot-tomless crevasses. What if I started to slip either left or right? Would my teammates be able to deter the pull of my dead weight?

Or would I end up in the bowels of Rainier's famous glaciers, disabled, strapped onto a sled, possibly having pulled in climbers on top of me?

Everyone was exhausted and relieved, several hours later, when we reached the Muir hut.

I was quickly unloaded and carefully carried inside by four of the guides. They laid me on top of my sleeping bag and unrolled the cocoon I had nestled in for the last four hours. It wasn't long before the agony and disappointment set in.

I had so wanted to reach the summit. I knew I could have made it, would have made it. But the pain was bad. If I moved even slightly, a searing red rocket of pain would shoot up my leg, through my torso, into my head, and down the other side, much like a pinball machine. The guides came to check on me regularly.

"How are you doing?" asked Link.

Robert Link is Native American, or so rumor has it. I hear that his parents are as pale as I am, but Link's dark coloring supports the rumor. His eyes are what set him apart, however—large dark eyes that reach back into his gentle soul. They have the depth of a high mountain lake, and that night all I saw in them was pain, my pain reflected in his compassion.

"I guess I won't be running in the race in Granville, Ohio, next week. I was really counting on it, having the whole family there for a reunion in the town where we were raised. I even designed the running outfits," I babbled, not sure I wanted to hear what he might have to say.

"I don't think so," he replied softly.

But I knew that even before he opened his mouth. His eyes said it all. I had never been hurt badly before, but I was now, for sure. The pain never let up, rolling from one end of my body to the other. The aspirin I had been given was useless.

Later, much to my chagrin, I had to go to the bathroom.

"You have two choices," I was told. "We can either bring in a pot, or a couple of these big strong boys can carry you to the outhouse."

I had always been so independent, never needing to rely on anyone. I could handle it myself, but not now, not this time. As I debated the pot versus the outhouse, I looked up and realized how much the people I was with wanted to help. For the very first time I realized that people need to be needed. I typically didn't allow much room for that in my life, but this time I was willing and thankful to be carried to the head.

Twenty-four hours later, I had survived the night without painkillers, and a sleeping bag was wrapped around my swollen and throbbing ankle, and I was loaded back on the litter. The weather had cleared, and it was safe to get me off the mountain. The only question was who would take me down. Four people were required. A climber would be roped to each corner of the sled in order to safely control the speed on the steep slopes leading back to the guide house.

Often, in the mountains, I am surprised by a side of humanity that doesn't regularly surface in city life. On the morning I was to be evacuated, six of my team members volunteered to give up their summit bid to help me out. It took three and a half hours to maneuver the sled and the bulk of my dead weight down the mountain.

Only once was I concerned. Less than an hour above Paradise Lodge, my porters eased up, knowing we were close. I felt the litter slide sideways and saw an overgrown fir looming ever closer. I shouted, "There's a tree. I'm afraid I might hit that tree," and I was quickly pulled back on line. The ceaseless pain I had experienced on the mountain was behind me. I was so happy to be going down.

Mount Rainier National Park, however, is far away from any large metropolitan area. On arriving at the base of the mountain, my best bet was to ride shotgun in a two-seater Triumph for the two-hour drive to Puyallup. What a strange-sounding name. One that I would never forget. My destroyed ankle bounced up and down as guide Skip Yowell drove. I winced as the pinball spasm returned, but I knew that a doctor would soon take care of my pain and discomfort.

The next day I woke up in a metal-sided bed in the Puyallup, Washington, hospital with a solid cast on my leg and a pin and a screw holding together the three shattered bones in my reconstructed ankle.

After a hearty dose of painkillers, I sat wondering how I could contact Roger. I didn't have to mull it over for very long. When the phone rang, I answered, "Evans Mountaineering."

"It's me, big shot," came Roger's voice over the line.

Then, I cried.

CHAPTER 3

Transition

In order to see the birds it is necessary
to become a part of the silence.
Robert Lynd (1879–1949)

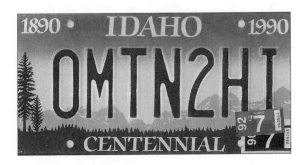

There is a strain, a big anxiety, when you know you have a life-threatening disease. The tension gets bigger when you think only your attitude can save you. You try to avoid any stress or confrontation. Yet every problem is magnified because your whole being is on edge, poised to not make a mistake that will spread the cancer unstoppably through your system, multiplying, destroying, and potentially killing that which you hold so dear—your life.

———■———

In my early twenties I was hired at Helga, a leading design firm in Los Angeles that specialized in couture clothing for women. It was my first real job, other than freelance work, in my chosen field. Even though I did very little designing, I felt as if I was truly in the world of high fashion. It was my sketches that revealed all the exciting new styles to prospective new clients, my body that often modeled them, and my hand that wrote the orders at out-of-town trunk shows. All the latest styles would travel with me in oversized trunks to specialty and department stores where, at in-store receptions, Helga's faithful customers could purchase from the entire line.

The doyen of the firm was Helga Erteszak, an older, distinguished woman with slicked-back hair, a road map of a face, and two five-carat diamonds on one finger. She used to say to me, "If you have your health, you have everything," and I used to look at her as if she was from Mars. I was young and invincible. But she would still remind me often, "You must mind your health. Without it you have nothing."

One of my duties as assistant designer was to fit Mrs. Erteszak's rich clientele and close friends in Helga Originals. All of these women were old enough to be my mother and, in many cases, old enough to be my grandmother. With one difference. Many of them had had breast cancer. In the closet of a dressing room next to the showroom, I would watch those women change into neatly tailored suits and extravagant gowns. I would notice with compassion, although no attachment, their breastless chests, which had been mutilated, leaving a maze of scars.

I had never seen the effects of a radical mastectomy before, but in the three years I was with Helga, I saw many. I would look into the sad faces of those ladies, offering what youthful radiance I could. But somehow I had felt immune, as if this particular condition was confined to a race of which I was not a part. Not once had I thought that I or anyone close to me would get breast cancer. And now, I had it. I couldn't believe that this was going to be me.

I felt like I had been hit by a meteorite that totally splintered my life. I was reminded of a childhood nightmare. The dream starts as a blank canvas, an empty space that is slowly filled by a rhythmic flow of energy, no specific form, just the easy, controlled movement of a mass. It is very peaceful and soothing, until suddenly, unexpectedly, it disrupts, shattering into a volcanic burst of light and power shooting out in all directions in frenetic disorder.

The nightmare had become real.

The same recurring questions ricocheted around my brain. How can I have cancer? Am I going to die? I am too young to die. What about Kilimanjaro? The climb I had planned would have to be put on hold. Would it ever happen? I love my husband, our house, and my career. I have been working so hard for my newest client, the Company Store, making good money. What will happen to my business?

Nothing. Everything would be put on hold, I realized after the shock subsided. The only important thing in my life at that moment was my health. Why, I have since wondered, do we have to get sick to learn that? So many years later, I finally realized that Helga was right.

In the fall of 1988, I had gotten a cold that developed into bronchitis, then I had temporarily lost my hearing. I'd ignored the fact that I was getting worse and worse and just popped pills and continued running and working, pushing forward with the hectic pace of my life. I wondered if that was the beginning of my cancer.

A year before my bout with bronchitis, I had started on the Fit or Fat diet, and I followed it religiously. I ate no salad dressings, no peanuts, no cheese, no avocados—all of which are satellite foods, orbiting out there on the forbidden periphery of what is low in fat and considered healthy, at least by the diet's creator, Covert Bailey. Before that my diet had not been exemplary. During the day I dined on fast food in wrappers, something that I could stock and eat on the run. No Big Macs or french fries; I drew the line somewhere. But this was not a well-balanced diet. Is that why I got cancer?

Dr. Campanale said, "You must not allow yourself to think negatively. You must focus all your energy on getting well and believe that you will. There is so much we don't know about breast cancer. But we do know that the statistics don't necessarily relate if you have the right attitude."

He said this just after telling me that the cancer had spread, that I was now a stage three (out of four), and that my chances for long-term survival had just dropped 50 percent.

How could I possibly maintain a good attitude? It was all so sudden and foreign and frightening. I felt trapped in the isolation of my illness. My friends and family were supportive, but they hadn't been through cancer. How could they truly understand?

The pain of the biopsy and subsequent surgery was nothing compared to the pain in my heart. I felt the burden of responsibility to get myself well again, to make the right decisions in terms of doctors and treatment, to think all the right thoughts. In my confusion and shock, it was a lot to bear.

After the results of the final tests were evaluated, Dr. Campanale looked me straight in the eye and added, "Once cancer takes hold of the body, it becomes a contest of wills."

Again, I thought about Dad, and I gazed down at the silver ID bracelet on my wrist. Charles W. Steele, it read beneath a fine web of scratches. I never took the bracelet off. It had been a gift from Mom to Dad long before I was born. I don't remember him wearing it. I had found it after he died in his top desk drawer, along with his favorite pens, an envelope of stamps, and pictures of us, the kids. I missed Dad. Was I going to see him again soon? Did I subconsciously will this to happen? "I'm not ready to die," I announced out loud, meaning it.

My focus became singular. I meditated, sitting on the floor cross-legged in the dark, trying desperately to free my mind of all the unpleasant thoughts that probed in the corners. I dug out my father's diaries and sought comfort and understanding in his "Temas" or ideas:

- One must live with the consequences of his acts.
- If there isn't justice in life, there is a sort of law of averages.
- Sacrifice and self-punishment bring perspective.
- Basic optimism (hope) and pessimism (fear) persist in the individual.
- The essential ingredient is the willingness to take a chance, to act on behalf of something beyond oneself.

- Any man can fight his own heroic battles within himself. And, if he thinks and acts the hero, he will like himself and life will not be a burden.
- A sense of sacrifice helps. A willingness to give to the other person at the expense of one's own interests; in other words, humility.
- One needs a balanced appreciation of his own importance and lack of importance. He must always remind himself that the ocean of life is vast and that there is always somebody better.
- Indispensable is a sense of humor (the mysterious absurdity of life must not get us down). Human nature is imperfect—that is why humor is so important.

It was hard to believe how rosy things could be one day and how bleak the next, but as Dad had known, it was the law of averages of life. What is, is. I would make the best of it. Somehow. I vowed to give every ounce of energy I had to the challenge that lay ahead.

In the bathroom, next to my sink, I hung my favorite Christmas present. It was a gift from our good friends Nancy and Steve Butler. Whenever I looked at it, it gave me strength. It was a pastel painting of the mountains in soft morning light with one regal evergreen in the foreground and the words: No Mountain Too High. That would become my sole focus. Two weeks later I even translated those words for the license plate of my Jeep: 0MTN2HI.

Because the holidays had arrived, we went out a few times, but it was tough. I could see my plight written in the faces of those around me, friends who were sympathetic but fearful for their own lives. I could hear their minds at work: "If this could happen to Laura. . . ." I even watched in horror as a good friend crossed the street to avoid me as if I were contagious. She later apologized, but facts were facts. Dad had once said, "No man's life is complete without his death." As humans we don't want to accept that.

New Year's Eve was particularly difficult. Normally I would have been excited, anxiously looking forward to what lay ahead, armed with my long list of resolutions and challenges for the coming year. Now there was only one thing on my list. GET WELL. But I knew it wouldn't be easy, that this would be the toughest year of my life. I knew it would take hard, focused work. And I suspected that I would be tested physically and mentally in most unpleasant ways—in ways, I was sure, I could not yet fathom. On that last day of 1989, I didn't want to think too much about what the new year would hold.

All of this was exceedingly hard on Roger. We had spent half our lives together, moving across the country and traveling around the world. With each new location, we had grown closer and relied more on each other. It was inconceivable that after the recent and unexpected loss of his mother, Roger would lose me, too. He struggled to maintain the internal strength that we would both need.

I reflected on easier times, when Roger and I first met. It had been twenty years earlier.

Roger walked into my life when I was managing a popular hamburger joint in Columbia, Missouri, one of several jobs I held while working my way through college. He was an admissions officer at Stephens, where I was studying fashion design. Lean and long at six-foot-three, 180 pounds, with a big bushy mustache, he definitely caught my eye. But after a brief conversation, I didn't see him again for three months. By then, I was cocktail waitressing at Jack's Coronado, one of the fancier restaurants in town.

He showed up with a buddy of his, had a quick drink, and left. I didn't think he really noticed me until he phoned later to ask if I would like to join him Friday night for dinner.

"A lady I work with has invited a few friends over for a dove dinner," he informed me. "Would you like to be my date?"

It took me about a half a second to answer. "Yes." Yes, yes, yes!

Friday night we went to the dinner. I had never eaten dove before, and after that first experience I vowed never to eat it again. There are too many small crunchy bones, I thought that night as I chomped them into the smallest possible pieces before swallowing.

I remember looking over at Roger's plate and seeing his little bird bones all neatly stacked in one corner. I even watched him, out of the corner of my eye, pull them from his mouth with his fingers.

I'll be damned if I'm going to stick my fingers in my mouth, I thought, not in front of Roger. He's definitely too good-looking.

Later that evening I regretted my decision. Down on my knees, I held the sides of the toilet bowl as I heaved. All this for a man? Actually, it's best that I'm throwing up, I reminded myself. God knows what those bones could do in my system.

A couple of months later, Roger stood on top of a checkered tablecloth in St. Louis and announced to a startled roomful of diners that he would like to make a special toast. Before I could react, Roger removed his leather loafer, filled it with beer, and spoke.

"I would like to make a toast to the most beautiful girl in the world," he grinned, brandishing his size twelve and a half beer mug. Now he had everybody's attention. "To Laura and to love." Gulp went the beer. And plunk went my heart.

Roger and I are "lifers," destined to be together forever. But now forever began to look a little too soon for comfort.

Roger had just spent much of December calling friends and hospitals for recommendations on doctors. We had narrowed it down to one in Idaho and two in San Francisco. We had lived in the Bay Area before moving to Sun Valley and felt more comfortable with the idea of my treatment taking place in a location that was familiar. Besides, a meeting with the oncologist in Boise had proved disappointing. I had gotten the distinct impression that this doctor hadn't even read my test results thoroughly. At some point in our brief conversation he had advised me "to carry on with my life as usual." Say what? Is it that simple to slip on a wig (that would be inevitable), slip back into the mainstream, and erase from my mind the fact that the next six months would very likely determine the rest of my life? As a response to his suggestion that he hook me up on chemotherapy right then and there, Roger and I flew to San Francisco for another opinion.

On the fourth day of the new year, Roger and I had a long, productive meeting with Dr. Kathleen Grant, an oncologist at Pacific Presbyterian Hospital. She came highly recommended, and we were pleased with her knowledge, quiet manner, and sincere concern. She was also well informed on my prognosis and had given considerable thought to what treatment I should consider.

"Although you have what is termed a garden variety, because it is fast growing and estrogen negative, it is more tenacious, more dangerous than your average breast cancer. Also the involvement of eleven malignant lymph nodes is a significant number. I feel for certain that you will need chemotherapy and radiation."

This came as no surprise, since we had already heard the same thing before. Many times. Yet, Dr. Grant's understated manner somehow made it easier to accept.

"Will that give me the best chance for long-term survival?" I wanted to know.

"Are there any other options that should be considered?" Roger asked.

"I would like to give you a thorough checkup before I make any final recommendations," she responded.

At our encouragement, Dr. Grant decided to move right along. She did needle biopsies on two small lumps in my neck (where had those come from?). Twice she hit a nerve, and it felt like someone was shooting burning sparklers up and down my arm. That was followed by a bone marrow biopsy. I felt like I was getting treatments in *One Flew over the Cuckoo's Nest.*

When the tests were complete and the results back, Dr. Grant recommended that we seriously consider a clinical test being offered at Pacific Presbyterian that would include intensive chemotherapy followed by a bone marrow transplant. Whether or not I opted for the bone marrow procedure, I would still need several months of outpatient chemo to ensure that I had no unexpected side effects to the drugs before being blasted with the heavier doses. Everything I read or heard mentioned how rough these drugs were. What she was proposing sounded horrible, but I knew I must view the drugs as medicines, as my one shot at getting well.

Also, I realized I wasn't the first one to go through this. Thousands of people had cancers worse than mine, and they mustered their will to live. My heart went out to these people as I became more involved in the realities and "cure" for the disease. I resolved to help out other cancer patients once (not if) I got through this. Several breast cancer survivors had talked to me shortly after I'd been diagnosed. It had made such a difference just seeing living, breathing members of the human race who had survived the hell I was now going through.

After my conversations with Dr. Grant, I thought about Kilimanjaro and how much I had looked forward to climbing it. Only three weeks earlier I had mentally set up a training schedule: more weights, more hikes, more yoga. Now there would be no Kilimanjaro. Not this year. Maybe never. It saddened me to think how long it had taken me to realize that I wanted to be a mountaineer and that now I might never get the chance.

I called Peter, who could only respond, "We'll climb it for you. You'll be back."

I knew I was tough, but my life had been turned upside down. I would not be carrying packs up Baldy. Instead I would be pumped with drugs that would do God-knows-what to my body.

But somewhere deep down I believed, had to believe, that I would be back someday in the mountains I had grown to love.

CHAPTER 4

Side Effects

What lies behind us and what lies before us are
tiny matters compared to what lies within us.

Ralph Waldo Emerson

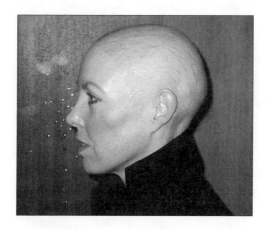

*I must pursue those ideals that I have wanted and wor-
shiped and kept at arm's length in lieu of more "important"
or impressive endeavors. To say I want to do something is
no longer sufficient. These are empty, meaningless words
that add a burden to an already heavy load.*

————————■————————

In February of 1990, I was in San Francisco for the second of
my three outpatient chemo treatments before entering the
hospital for the clinical trial. The first chemo treatment was per-
manently etched in my mind since it had been administered on
my forty-first birthday. But the drugs and the grueling side effects
were made bearable through the generosity of our friends Barney
and Diana Upton. They opened up their arms and beautiful
home on the hillside in Sausalito, just across the bay from San
Francisco, for my three monthly visits.

I arrived at the Uptons the evening before my early morning
appointment. Looking out their vast expanse of glass at the San
Francisco Bay, I thought of the times I had windsurfed and
sculled on those waters. I thought, somewhat wistfully, of the
five-mile race on Angel Island, my fastest time ever—seven-
minute miles—and the guy behind me thanking me for pulling
him through.

All that was history. Now I could barely move. The side
effects of the drugs had started showing up only two days after
my first dose of chemotherapy. My upper body had become so

racked with aches and pains that even with relaxants I couldn't sleep.

A week before my trip, determined not to stay in bed, I had tried to go for a walk, but my thumbs were so arthritic I couldn't put on my coat. It was too heavy, too awkward for me to contort my body into. I had collapsed in tears, destroyed by my own weakness. I'd even had to ask Roger to help me put on my own socks and twist the cap off a bottle of mineral water. I could no longer wear sweatshirts or any shirts with buttons. I could not lift my forearms higher than my elbows, and my shoulders were racked with pain.

Dr. Grant said she had never before heard of aching, swelling joints as a side effect of chemotherapy. An arthritis specialist went so far as to say I had rheumatoid arthritis, a totally separate illness. I reminded them both that I had been running six pain-free miles a day prior to my diagnosis and the administration of the drugs.

To combat the increasing swelling, Prednisone, a steroid, had been prescribed. Although I loathed the idea of more drugs in my system, because of the Prednisone I at least could move around and sleep a little.

I slowly showered and changed before the Uptons returned from work. I knew that a small dinner party was planned for that evening, and I wanted to give myself plenty of time to prepare. My wig sat on the bathroom counter as I put on mascara and rouge. Anything to make me look well. Standing there, I inspected the shape of my head, turning it from side to side. I realized how few people know the shape of their heads, how it protrudes out in the back and slopes down to the neck. As I inspected my skull, I thought about the few short weeks it had taken to go bald.

I had known the hair would go. And to lessen the trauma when it did, I'd gone to my hairdresser and had him chop it off.

The ponytail was sitting in a baggie at home, as if sometime in the future I could reattach it. What hair was left hadn't lasted long. I kept willing it to stay on my head, but it had fallen out anyway. Countless hairs littered my pillow and my face and ended up in my food. Then one night, when I went to rearrange my bangs, they came off in my hand.

I had stood in front of the bathroom mirror, with Roger watching in horror, as I pulled out clumps of hair at a time, making a nest in my open palm.

"How can you do this to me?" Roger had asked.

"I'm not doing this to you." I had replied.

There, reflected in the mirror, was the most visible aspect of my illness. The large unframed eyes that stared back from the glass were those of someone acutely ill. Gone was the illusion that this was all a bad dream; it was now a painful reality.

But we had to laugh or else we would only cry. The day I bought the first of three wigs, we howled. It was a huge mane of fluffy red curls, a cross between Ann-Margret and Little Orphan Annie. Roger's reaction was, "You look like a hooker," which, considering how unsexy I felt, was somewhat of a compliment.

Roger also referred to me affectionately as Gandhi, but I thought I looked more like Leonard Nimoy.

Without the wig and without my eyebrows and pubic hairs, which had also taken a hike, I pointed out to Roger that my current condition gave a whole new meaning to the word *naked*.

I ended my reminiscing when I heard Diana drive into the garage, and I quickly slipped my wig back on my head. I went out to greet her.

"It's miserable out there," Diana informed me as she dropped a couple shopping bags onto her bed.

"It wasn't raining very hard when I got here," I mentioned. "It actually seems rather soothing when you're on the inside looking out."

"I just hope our guests don't have a problem getting here," she fretted. "They are due to arrive in an hour. And I'm worried about Barney. He's driving from the airport."

Thirty minutes later the storm escalated. Outside the bedroom window, I could hear branches slamming against the sides of the house. Harsh sleet drummed on the roof, and the lights flickered, then went out.

"Shit," I heard Diana react. "Shit!"

"Can I do anything?" I offered.

"No. Stay where you are. I'll go find some candles."

Minutes later, Diana delivered a candle to my room. As she hurried around lighting up other parts of the house, I glanced in the mirror, checking myself out. Spooky, I thought, and suddenly I chuckled. Unable to resist, I took off my wig and held the candle under my chin. Bella Lugosi would have been proud.

This ought to take Diana's mind off the current but not significant disaster, I thought as I tiptoed out of the bedroom into the pitch dark of the hallway. I could hear her footsteps coming down the stairs, and I had to stifle my laughter.

"Oooooooo . . ." I let out as she eased off the bottom step.

"Aaaaaaahhhhhh!" she shrieked.

When she realized it was me, we both stood there in the dark laughing so hard we almost wet our pants.

More typically, at my home among the snow-covered mountains, day after uneventful day dragged by slowly. I would often sit in the oversized chair in the corner of our living room with my feet propped on its matching ottoman. Beside me would be stacks of cancer books and my diary. But instead of reading or writing I would find myself staring out the window up at the ski mountain, thinking of all the people I knew, my husband included, who were out there having a good time.

I wanted that again. *There is so much to live for, so many things I enjoy,* I reinforced in my mind as I steeled my resolve to make whatever changes were necessary to get well. I would coax out of my life any old habits that had taken their toll in the name of duty or friendship. I intended to put into perspective the opinions of those who knew and loved me. I would try very hard to make only decisions that worked best for me.

But it wasn't easy. There were times, sitting in that chair, that I felt suspended in space, not in any concrete reality. I couldn't deny my illness, nor could I live it every minute of every day. But it was always there, leering, hanging around my neck like some ominous albatross. The spark that had previously emanated from my very core was gone.

The nights were awful. I would close my eyes and visualize shooting my disease and stabbing it, rolling over it, stomping on it, and catapulting it into the sea. In my mind's eye, I would watch it get eaten up by huge fish that swam far out into the ocean.

Then I would lie there wide awake listening to Roger's ragged breathing, afraid to move because of the incessant pain and afraid to sleep for fear I would wet the bed. And when I did have to go to the bathroom, I would have to roll out of bed slowly and inch my way to the toilet, where I would have to pee standing up, for I could not bend my knees, even slightly, without discomfort. The prospect of squatting on a toilet was inconceivable.

And there was always so much prodding and poking and pricking and pain. Blood had to be drawn regularly to determine the state of my white blood cell count, which constituted my immune system. But because of the toxicity of the chemo, my veins refused to cooperate. They would roll over and hide or just refuse to bleed. On one particularly memorable visit to the doctor's office, the nurse, having decided to give my arms a break, pricked four different fingers before drawing blood. That was also the day that fluid was removed from my arthritic knees and a one-hour IV was administered in hopes of relieving some of the discomfort.

As I got closer to the in-hospital stay, the days got tougher. The dread of spending six to eight weeks in a bacteria-free bubble and the fear of what would and could happen in there were overwhelming. We spent many of those last days on the phone with the insurance company, trying to convince them that this clinical trial could, in fact, save my life. After much discussion, they finally came through, if only partially, agreeing to pay for the chemotherapy and hospital stay but not the bone marrow harvest or transplant. I found that rather amusing, since without the bone marrow I couldn't survive.

I spent hours deciding what I would take with me, what little things would bring me some sort of comfort. I selected pictures of Roger and me, several good (noncancer) books, a yet-to-be-started needlepoint project, my favorite videos (including *A Fish Called Wanda*), some new coral-colored Victoria Secret's pajamas, and a twelve-inch battery-operated plastic dancing flower with bold yellow sunglasses and a matching guitar.

We were invited to one last farewell party. Although I appreciated the gesture and ultimately wanted to be with my friends, the party promised to be tough. Seeing my contemporaries so healthy and vibrant would be a torturous reminder of the gap between us and the long hard road that lay ahead for me. Yet when we walked into our neighbor's house, everyone was wearing three-inch buttons that read, "We Love You, Laura." What more could I ask?

Two days before our departure for San Francisco, the weather turned gorgeous, but time was slipping away. I found myself frequently, suddenly, and unexpectedly on the verge of tears, as if my body knew, instinctively, that it would miss all that was being left behind. The sunshine, the fresh air, the walks. I knew I would miss Sun Valley, my office studio, our house, our friends, the smell of the pine trees in the mountains.

The mountains. Would I ever scale them again? How long ago it now seemed when I first started climbing, when I first woke up in a field of white with the stars twinkling overhead and a round ball of light beckoning me higher. "Come join me," the man in the moon seemed to be saying. "There are answers up here that can be found nowhere else. Come join me."

On Rainier, I learned what mountaineer Rene Dumal meant when he said,

> You cannot stay on the summit forever, you have to come down again. So why bother in the first place?
>
> Just this: What is above knows what is below, but what is below does not know what is above.
>
> One climbs, one sees. One descends, one sees no longer, but one has seen.
>
> There is an art of conducting oneself in the lower regions by the memory of what one saw higher up.
>
> What one can no longer see, one can at least still know.

In the mountains, I had learned about priorities and interdependence. I had learned about the body's and mind's ability to push beyond. I had learned that the bond of friendship forged in a life-threatening situation is stronger than any other. I had learned that when it is all said and done, we really are all equal. In so many ways, I had learned about love and respect, for my peers and myself, for those of us who had the courage and strength to follow the path of our dreams.

———————■———————

CHAPTER 5

Rainier Revisited

What is life? It is the flash of a firefly in the night. It is the breath of a buffalo in the wintertime; it is the little shadow which runs across the grass and loses itself in the sunset.

Last words of Crowfoot

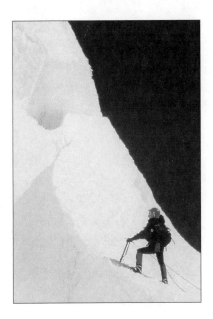

*I want to digest all the diverse elements that enter my life
and to understand the energy, the beauty, the interaction—
to feel that this life has touched mine and I it.*

———————————■———————————

We had been up for nearly five hours and had been moving
for almost three. Although it was barely light out, the
cloudless and windless sky held promise of a good day. It had
taken my body a full sixty minutes to get used to the idea of func-
tioning at the rude hour of 3:00 A.M., but I was now awake. Wide
awake.

We were traversing one of the many ice bridges that provide
temporary and uneasy travel across Rainier's legendary crevasses.
Annually, climbers get injured or swallowed up by these foreboding
gashes in the snow and ice. They are clearly nothing to mess
with. You want to get across them as fast and as carefully as possible. After the first bridge, I had found myself calculating the
weight on the rope.

*Five people, let's see, two women averaging 150 each (includ-
ing our light packs), three guys at around 180 each, plus their
fifteen- to twenty-pound packs. . . .* A lot of weight. I knew that the
route on the upper mountain changed often because certain
snow crossings were no longer considered safe. I hoped that the
900 or so pounds of climbers tied together on my rope wouldn't
put one of these to the test.

The ice bridge we were currently on was one of the scariest I had seen. Even in the dim early morning light, the foreboding jaws of the crevasse exposed hundreds of feet of ice ending somewhere in the center of the earth. I focused my eyes on the narrow one-foot trail in front of me, placing each step carefully, making sure the knife points on my crampons dug in. Ten feet and I was home free, or at least I was out of immediate danger of falling. No one, however, was out of harm's way until we had all crossed safely. One slip from anyone, and we could all end up down there together in that frozen tomb. I gripped my ice ax more firmly, proceeding one careful step at a time.

Ahead of me, I could see Peter Whittaker's outline. I could imagine the tension between his shoulder blades. Five or six years earlier, in a freak accident, a centuries-old chunk of ice had broken loose and buried part of Peter's rope team forever in the frigid depths of Rainier. It was a tragedy for which he wasn't responsible but would never forget.

Just as I neared the open field of snow, preparing to let out a sigh of relief, I heard John, who was tied to the rope directly behind me, mutter something.

"What?" I replied, not understanding what he said.

"There's a crampon," he repeated.

A crampon? I looked down at my boots. The crampon that had been strapped to my left foot only minutes earlier was missing. *Oh, shit!*

Peter also was looking down at my boots. "Laura, go back and get it."

"Go back and get it?" I asked, disbelieving.

"Go back and get it," he said again with some urgency in his voice.

Slowly I started to walk backward toward the center of the ice bridge.

"No, Laura. Turn around." Peter said patiently.

Turn around? On one foot of hard-packed snow with only one crampon?

I knew he wasn't kidding, although I briefly hoped as much. Cautiously I turned, putting more weight on the steel spikes on my right foot. How did I get talked into clip-on crampons, anyway? Never, ever again. In the past, I had used the strap-on kind. Even though they took a little longer to weave back and forth over the boot, they definitely were more secure. "I don't believe this," I muttered to myself.

After six heart-thumping steps, I bent down and retrieved my faulty equipment, then made my way slowly back to safety. Once the whole rope team had made it across, I eased into a snow bank, clipped the crampon back on, and cinched its one strap as tight as it would go. For the rest of our eight-hour day on the upper mountain, I worried that it would come off again.

This was my second time on Rainier since I had shattered my ankle. It had taken me two long years of casts, crutches, and physical therapy to build back enough strength to attempt the mountain again. But I had to. It was mountain one, Laura zip.

Now, with any luck at all and no more mishaps, the score would be Laura two, Rainier one.

I thought about Dad, who was a big part of why I was here. He was the first and only one who had ever called me dogged. I had been eight years old. I think in many ways I had wanted to be my father's son. I would troop after him on his forays into the woods to dig up trees to add to the ones he had already lovingly handpicked and planted on our property. My face flush with exertion, plump little arms and legs pumping, pistonlike, as fast as they could, I would keep pushing forward in a determined effort to keep up. Dad would always smile back at me, pleased with my tenacity, offering encouragement.

"You're dogged, Laura," Dad announced one evening. "I like that."

But I didn't like it. I just stared at him, mute. How could Dad think I was like a dog? Years later when I finally learned that *dogged* meant persistent, I inwardly smiled at Dad's accurate assessment. I was dogged. If I wanted something, somehow I'd get it. I believed that I could do anything or have anything I wanted if I was willing to work hard enough to get it.

Because of Dad and my desire to get his attention, I had become the jock in the family. My brother, who was older, tried, but he was really far more suited to academia. Both Lisa and Martha, my youngest and middle sisters, were active, but I was practically obsessed with sports. I joined the swim team, logging three hours a night, four days a week in the pool. I would stroke lap after endless lap just so on a Saturday afternoon in August I could see Dad's proud and smiling face as I stood, after the finish of the race, to receive my blue ribbon.

And here I was on Mount Rainier, closing in on my second successful summit to fully erase any residual fear, any trepidation lingering after my ankle injury. Only this time, the climbing experience was very different. Around my neck was a thirty-inch cord that attached to a six-inch red plastic tube. Inside were Dad's ashes. He had died two weeks earlier. As devastated as I was, I thought the climb would be good for me, might somehow remove me from the immediacy of my sorrow.

And I thought Dad would be pleased. He had requested near the end that my sister Lisa and I split up his ashes and distribute them over the Colorado mountains where Lisa lived and over the San Francisco Bay where I was living. Although it tore me apart to reach into the plastic bag and pull out fragments of bone and ash, I knew, being the adventurer that he was, that Dad would smile at the idea of a trip to the top of Rainier with his oldest daughter. Dad would once again be at the finish line for me, only this time smiling from afar.

Exhausted and sweaty, we made the summit six hours after we had set out. I contemplated what a bittersweet victory it was as I tossed Dad's ashes into the wind.

How I would miss his humble but educated wisdom! I had reread an excerpt from his diary just before this trip, and the words echoed in my mind.

> *I must not set myself upon a pedestal, and when I fail to reach my high ideals to worry about it. I must take myself as I am. I am only human, so instead of worrying when I seem to be below par, I'll realize that I'm no exception, but that I have every intention of building on the foundation I have already in the ways possible. I must look at life and note that it could be worse. We should live life to the full, making the most of our possibilities. The more we expend ourselves constructively, the more we live, the more we fulfill or carry out our role in the context of nature— some of the loneliness is dissipated, particularly when we reach others. In the very process of making a sacrifice, one attacks his greatest enemy, his ego.*

I would try my best.

I didn't socialize much on that climb, nor did I experience the elation I had two years earlier when I first crested Rainier's crater rim. At the time, I was the happiest person on the face of the earth, having achieved what I'd been unable to do on my first attempt. I had confronted my fears and climbed back on the horse. The trip was so different this time. I was still proud of my achievement, but it was overshadowed with sadness. I opted not to join the team in the bar of the Paradise Inn, normally the first stop off the mountain. I knew the bar would be packed with stinky bodies, rosy cheeks, big smiles, and lots of bottles of Bud. But not for me, not this time.

I was glad I had returned to the mountains. I enjoyed the intense quiet of climbing. All ears straining for unusual and unwelcome sounds, like the ground shifting underfoot. The acute awareness of one's own heart and lungs and muscles that are being tested to the max. The powerful embrace of nature, reflected in the guiding light of the stars and moon and the warmth of the early morning sun after hours of bone-chilling darkness. The soft cushion of snow on much-welcomed breaks and the ever-changing nuances of the surrounding peaks, dark and ominous before sunrise, then suddenly bright and inviting.

Although I couldn't bring myself to join the others in the bar, there was a warm spot in my heart for all of them. We had been out there together, helping one another stay alive and mentally focused. I also had an increasing amount of respect for all the guides at Rainier Mountaineering. They had made climbing a major part of their lives and unselfishly shared their love of the mountains with the rest of us flatlanders.

I knew I would be back again. What I didn't know, at the time, was what a difficult road it would be getting there.

CHAPTER 6

Isolation

The difference between loneliness and solitude is your perception of who you are alone with and who made the choice.

Anonymous

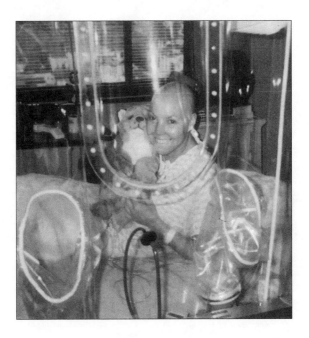

I broke down in an airport once in the middle of a long hall-way—in tears, shaken, shaking, without the will or energy to move my feet one more painful step. I was only vaguely aware of the helpless looks on the faces of those around me. Somehow I knew then, as I know now, that this would be a solitary battle. That each step I took would be through the sheer power of my will—regardless of how battered it would become.

———■———

I lay awake in my hospital bed, staring at the white walls. A year ago I had been looking up at the green nylon roof of a tent, feeling as if I had the cat by the tail, oblivious to the fact that life can change so quickly. It was hard to imagine that this body in this bed was the same one that had summited Mount Rainier several times. Thoughts of previous climbs were drowned out by the labored breathing of the woman asleep in the bed ten feet from mine, separated by a sheet posing as a curtain. I knew she, too, had cancer and was taking chemo. I could smell it, feel it, see it in her eyes when she was awake and the sheet was pulled aside. Fear secreted from her body the way sweat once did from mine, but it was mingled with hope and, I sensed, purpose. We had both elected to be here, to rid our bodies of the invasive demon that was threatening to take over our lives.

Beyond the walls of our room, I could hear the restless quiet of the darkened ward, the moans, an occasional cough, the retching of someone down the hall. Sleep was elusive as I contemplated what lay ahead. I had first heard about the clinical test I was about to undergo from my oncologist, Dr. Kathleen Grant. She had explained it to me in early January when we had first discussed the severity of my diagnosis.

"Your chances of getting cancer again are great, and if it does recur, we don't know how to treat it effectively," she had informed me, in her quiet, straightforward manner.

I didn't like what she had to say, but I respected her candor. Of the many doctors with whom I had spoken, she was the first to explain my situation clearly.

"What are my options?" I had asked, swallowing deeply.

"There is a clinical test. You would be a candidate for it. It involves intensive, high-dose chemotherapy followed by a bone marrow transplant." She described the treatment in layperson's terms: two miserable months in the hospital in an isolated, bacteria-free room being fed all liquids, food, and antibiotics intravenously. There would be nausea, hair loss, weakness, and increased susceptibility to serious infections, but ultimately a greater chance of surviving cancer for good.

I had stared at Dr. Grant in disbelief. Was she really recommending that I do this? I flashed on a cartoon I had recently seen that depicted a doctor talking to a patient. The caption read, "I want you to cut out red meat, alcohol, smoking, sex, and sports. Then we'll treat you for depression." What Dr. Grant had in mind for me certainly sounded depressing.

"What would you do," I had asked, "if you were me?"

"I would opt for the bone marrow transplant," she had responded after only a moment's hesitation. "It is the best chance you have for long-term survival."

Eventually I came to realize that she was right, the experimental protocol was my only viable alternative.

Consequently, three months after that conversation, I was lying in a hospital bed dreading the following day, when my roommate would be my roommate no longer. In the morning I would be escorted to my "cell," a six-by-nine-foot cubicle the size of a closet. There I would live for weeks, maybe months, with no human touch, until either I or the cancer was destroyed. Over the previous couple of days, in between tests and the insertion of my chest catheter, I had peeked into the other occupied laminair air flow rooms. I had seen the eyes of the occupants, blank and staring. An occasional smile would translate: "Yes, I'm glad I'm in here. No, it isn't fun. But yes, I will survive."

I clung to that thought. This was my one chance to save my life. As miserable as it would be, I could handle it. I knew I could handle anything for a short period of time. What's a couple of months compared to a lifetime? But I still couldn't sleep.

First light brought the nurse. "It's time."

Already? Oh shit. After being thoroughly cleansed, I followed the stark white shoes and uniform of my warden down the hall to the sterile room. I proceeded slowly, moving each foot inches at a time, trying to delay what was inevitable, savoring my last moments of freedom. I imagined this was what it felt like going to prison, walking down the long corridor past the other cells, knowing there was one with your name on it at the end, not aware of all that awaited you but certain it would be unpleasant. When we reached the door, she stepped aside. "There you go."

I stepped into the void, suddenly overwhelmed by fear, feeling its tendrils wrap around my very being, tightening its grasp. I turned to face my jailer.

"Don't lose it on me now," she responded, looking at the frozen, horrified look on my face. Her voice echoed from a world away. Somewhere in my subconscious, I recalled a passage I had once read: "Victims are not victims of the world they see; they are victims of the way they see the world." This was it. I might as well make the best of it.

I began to make myself at home. On the wall next to the mirror that hung over the sink I taped a calendar. On the metal cabinet beside the bed, next to my book and numerous magazines, I placed a large magic marker, which I planned to use every night, crossing off another day with a big *X*. Each mark would bring me that much closer to recovery and release. Above the plastic pan into which I would vomit, I tacked my "Hazards Exist" photo-poster, a shot of me skiing taken by my friend Nancy Hongola one week before I was diagnosed. In the picture I was radiant, happy, healthy, smiling at the camera. After using the throw-up dish, which I was told would be frequently, I could raise my head and look up at the wonderful life of the other me, a life I could surely get back. On my pillow sat Gordo, a stuffed bear of considerable heft, with whom I would snuggle in lieu of my husband. My yellow plastic dancing flower stood smiling behind the small cassette player on the night stand. This bright sunflower would be my partner for one song a day, if I could last that long before collapsing weak and exhausted onto the mattress.

The massive doses of chemo were administered, and within days most of my time was spent in bed. The bed was pushed up against a clear plastic window, close to the plastic sleeves into which the nurses put their arms to check on my chest catheter, into which flowed all my life-sustaining fluids. I had no sense of time. My days were not regulated by meals or appointments. I listened to the radio, worked on a needlepoint landscape, and once in a while watched a video. At night I fell asleep with the gentle nudge of Ativan and the soothing cassette sounds of surf and thunderstorms. In the mornings I awoke to the first hazy glow of the sun and the precious patch of green landscape framed by my hospital window. From almost the moment I entered my new residence, I longed to walk through that park, to smell the earth and grass and flowers, to hear the leaves rustle overhead and feel the wind caress my hair. The out-of-doors had become my home, my sanctuary, where I found peace. Sadly, though, I was separated from it by glass and intravenous tubing and cancer. Staring out the window, I vowed to walk through that park. One day.

Within the first week after having received the intensive chemo, my bone marrow was dripped through the catheter into my bloodstream. It had been extracted several weeks earlier, as I slept, by three doctors who used oversized needles to remove the marrow from my hip area. I was left with fifty or so round scars dotting my bum. It would take weeks, maybe months, for the white cells taken from my bones to rebuild enough to counteract the damage done by the drugs.

My family and friends came to visit. Many of them, through a blood drive Roger organized, had given red blood cells or platelets at the lab upstairs. They felt they should at least come down and make sure I was well enough to receive their donation. I greatly appreciated my friends' gesture, but their visits were often hard on me. Before going into the hospital I had been hurting physically and emotionally, but I was still, in a sense, well. In the expressions of those who came calling, though, there was no escaping the truth. I was very sick. Through the plastic, I could feel their fear and discomfort as they kept their distance, not coming too close to the thin, clear wall that separated them from me, them from a life-threatening illness. I could sense sorrow and pity directed at me and at Roger. I felt it in the arms encased in the plastic sleeves that would, on occasion, reach in tentatively to give me a hug. I saw it in my own eyes, which stared blankly back out of the mirror, frozen in a puffy bald head perched atop a body that no longer functioned as it used to.

Nonetheless, I looked forward to these visits, to seeing the faces that were a reminder of happier times and the assurance, somehow, of more good times to come. And I never lost sight of the love—in Roger's frequent visits and in my sisters', who left their families and traveled halfway across the country, and in my dear friend Mary Brent, who came every night after work or dinner and held my hand with the synthetic glove, even when I was asleep, willing me back to her world.

Mom flew out for a two-week visit, lavishing me with parental affection and concern. I was happy to see my mother, but I knew how very hard it was for her to see me sick and hurting and not be able to hold me. She would show up at the hospital about three in the afternoon.

"Hi, Mom," I would greet her cheerfully, no matter how bad I felt.

"Hi, dear. How are you doing?" Mom would ask as she pressed her face against the little plastic window that curved into my room.

"Okay," I would chuckle. Mom usually stopped at El Matador on Fillmore Street, two blocks from the hospital, for a couple of margaritas to brace herself for her visit. Seeing her slightly tipsy face mushed into the window of my bubble struck me as funny. *Whatever it takes,* I thought. *I wouldn't mind a margarita myself.*

"Children aren't supposed to die before their parents," she would remind me for the hundredth time.

"I'm not going to die, Mom. I'm going to be okay," I would reassure her and me at the same time.

"I know, dear, but I hate to see you suffer so much," she would say, swiping at tears. Her words were yet another reminder of how hard my situation was on everyone who knew me.

Cards came in from across the country, from all the neighborhoods where Roger and I had once lived. The support from so many people we knew reinforced in my mind that I would have to be tough and fight as hard as I could, for me and for them. Friends from southern California wrote:

When we first heard that you had cancer, we were angry. Angry that a disease could try to take the life of someone who loves living so much. Then our anger turned to frustration that we might not be able to help.

Laura, you're a fighter. We've always admired you for that. You're also a winner, and we know if anyone can beat cancer through sheer determination, you will.

We want you to know that we are pulling for you all the way. Enclosed is a small gold boxing glove charm. Please wear it to remind yourself that we're in this fight with you and we're expecting you to win!

Several buddies from Sun Valley decided to cheer me up. They flew to San Francisco and arrived at the hospital en masse, all smiles, as if anticipating a party. Shortly after they had descended on my alcove, a bouquet of balloons arrived, and somewhere out of the middle popped a man dressed up as a cross between a waiter and a clown. Dramatically swinging his arm in an arch, he announced, "This is from all your friends who put you in there."

"Excuse me?" I queried. "All my friends who put me in here?"

For all his instant bravado, Mr. Clown-Waiter was clearly uncomfortable. I got the distinct impression that someone had neglected to inform this young rookie that his evening's entertainment would be directed at someone in a transparent bubble. This was probably a part-time job, taken on for a little extra money and maybe a few kicks. Not this night, however.

Trying to atone for his shaky start, my jester began to sing. "You must have been a beautiful baby," he began in a clear, if not strong, voice.

Bad choice, I thought. *I should leave this poor kid alone,* my good angel urged. *But I get no chances to be ornery in here,* responded my bad angel. *Sorry, I can't resist.* With that I whipped off my turban and pumped my legs up and down. When the young singer mustered up the nerve to look my way to see what had generated the laughter, he found himself looking at what appeared to be a female Baby Huey, an adult-sized, bald-headed infant. I had puffed up in the hospital much like a blowfish, the high caloric diet adding thirty pounds of fluid to my normally trim frame. So indeed, I looked the part.

That was the end of my singing telegram and probably that kid's last night on the job.

As the days wore on, the strain of my circumstances increased. I missed the simple pleasures in life. Eating, for instance. I relished the thought of being able to put something in my mouth other than a toothbrush. Instead of the juicy first bite of a fresh piece of swordfish or the satisfying, fragrant bouquet of a fine wine, all I tasted were the medicines that permeated my body. I lived with the constant smell of rubber and plastic from my IV tubes and the odd odor of the clear wall by my bed and the spit-up tub where I vomited. My skin was pallid. I felt, at times, as if all the plastic and tubing and drugs were turning me into wax, the next exhibit at Madame Tussaud's museum.

I became totally dependent on the nursing staff, which was both reassuring and scarier than hell. Because bone marrow patients are in the hospital for such a long period of time, the nurses walk a fine line between becoming emotionally involved with people in their care and viewing them strictly as more patients. The isolation necessitates that the nurses provide a certain amount of emotional support. For the most part, the men and women who cared for me were both professional and sympathetic. They tended to my discomfort as best they could. The staff even provided me with plastic-arm hugs in the middle of the night, when I lay alone shivering, unable to hold back the tears or the fear that I might never get well again.

But competent people had their counterparts in incompetence. My head nurse, for instance, readily admitted that she did everything with three-quarters' effort. She explained that it leaves more time to do more things—at three-quarters' effort, of course. This was most evident when medicines didn't show up as scheduled. In the outside world I wouldn't have been as concerned, but in my locked-up and beaten-down state, my survival was at issue. Some medical assistants lacked skills and experience. When they labored over my ministrations, I would burrow into my bedclothes and pray. What if they pushed the wrong button, inadvertently giving me the incorrect dose? I was painfully aware that the catheter tube ran awfully close to my heart.

The chemotherapy drugs that transfused my system had quickly demolished my white blood cells, leaving me vulnerable to all the bacteria residing in my system. Phlegm clogged my throat, and I suffered piercing pains in my side, my body racked with incessant coughing. There was nothing left in my system to throw up except the foamy white lining of my lungs, which reminded me of shaving cream as it flowed from my wretched insides into the plastic pan. The doctors ran test after test, pumping me with a variety of antibiotics, trying to save my life. One drug, in particular, which the nurses nicknamed shake-and-bake, was my least favorite. While on it, I would become feverish, tearing off everything but my flimsy nightgown, then seconds later feel chilled to the bone, unable to get warm under layers of blankets.

On bad days I stared forlornly at the calendar on the wall, at all the empty days and meaningless Xs, afraid I would never leave that room, womb, tomb. But I searched out the healing white light in the hollow warehouse of my mind and clung to the faint but distinct vibes, the soft echo of my own voice, "You will be okay. This, too, shall pass. You will be well again."

My immune-deficient body was unable to ward off infection, and I became consumed with a high fever. My battered lungs filled with fluid. I could feel the gentle hands of death cradling me, lifting me up. During that time I understood that I was no longer afraid. Death was a release. It would be so easy to close my eyes, leaving behind the pain and discomfort, the worry, the struggle of life. I could just float away into a pleasant, faraway place.

But through the haze of my fever, I saw, beyond my window, the distorted, anguished faces of my husband, mom, sister, and dear friends. I saw their alarm and wanted to comfort them, to tell them death was not so bad, to let them know it would be okay. But they wouldn't understand. They were on the other side of the line. They only knew that they loved me and needed me, as I needed them.

As easy as it would have been in my debilitated state, I couldn't die. I couldn't leave all those who had pulled so hard for me, who were counting on me, who were relying on my strength and their faith. I clung to the life I loved and the sure knowledge that I would get well. One day, I would get well. It wasn't my time.

When the fever finally broke, I thought more about death. What an elusive thing it is. What an elusive thing we have made it, hiding it under sheets, behind closed doors, under our breaths. Perhaps it doesn't really exist. Perhaps no one really dies. Maybe they go on extended vacations. I smiled weakly, knowing that I had been offered that ticket. What a fine destination it had seemed, free of care and suffering and effort, but so hard on those left behind. All those who had not held this ticket didn't know how it felt—so weightless in your hand. For the first time in my life I understood the peace and release that come with death. I also began to understand the value of living in that same way, without the weight of the world on my shoulders, feeling a gentle acceptance and appreciation for myself and others and the process of life-death-life itself.

CHAPTER 7

Release

Experience is a hard teacher because
she gives the test first, the lesson after.

Vernon Law

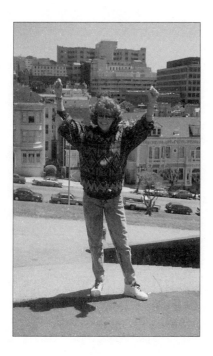

Cancer has caused me to look at the world through new eyes: my old eyes are clear in the knowledge that I had pushed the boundaries too hard and too far. And now, my young eyes are confused and wondering at the pain and suffering that are an integral part of growing up. I do realize what a big role attitude plays in the healing process, and I am forced for the first time to accept death as a natural part of the life process.

———■———

Seven weeks after I entered the laminair air flow room, I stood on the metal steps of the fire escape leading down from the fifth floor of the Pacific Presbyterian Hospital. On my head, like a jester's crown, was the blue paper mask that generally sat over my nose and mouth, the safety net between me and all the germs lurking in the air waiting to attack my weakened immune system. I forgot it was there. The solitude of the confinement of the last weeks slipped away. I was free again. I wasn't free to leave the hospital, but I was outside filling my lungs with fresh, sweet air, feasting my eyes on the glorious green lawn, trees, and, bushes, filling my senses with the sweet sounds of birds, the rustle of the wind. In that moment, atop a series of harsh metal steps, I was as happy and grateful as I have ever been. The bone marrow transplant had been a success. Through weeks of waiting, my white blood cell count had increased little by little, until now my immune system was strong enough that I could live outside my bubble.

Two days later, in the outpatient room designed to wean me from the laminair air flow room and allow my body time to get used to a nonsterile environment, I developed viral pneumonia. I was subjected to a series of uncomfortable tests, which produced no conclusive results. Long metal tubes were stuck into my nose, down my throat, and into my lungs. Liquids were sprayed into my mouth. I couldn't breathe. I could think only of poor Michael Palin in *A Fish Called Wanda,* with french fries up his nose and an apple in his mouth. I had nothing to divulge. Why was I being tortured?

A metal IV dispenser rack, much like a sturdy coat tree, was installed next to my bed, between me and the chair where my husband often sat, concerned, trying to act cheerful. "You'll be out of here soon." I hoped he was right. I seemed to get sick, then well, then sick. I so wanted to be well again, for good. On the metal rolling rack were bottles of antibiotics, liquids, food, and morphine. Each was connected to a separate computer, which monitored the dosages that dripped through the tubes into my chest catheter. In my nose were oxygen tubes. I grew weaker. I rested my head on the right side so I could transport myself into the land of the aspens in the mural-sized photo my friend Roy Toma had sent me. I speculated that he must have shot the aspens very early in the morning. The light backlit the leaves, waking them up, unfolding their beauty to the world.

I had to go to the bathroom but didn't have the strength to lift myself out of bed.

Finally out of necessity I did, carefully rolling the hundred-pound rack behind me. The toilet was three feet past the bed in its own small room next to a matching sink. While in isolation, I had longed for a real toilet, tiring of the port-a-potty with its plastic bag, which I would have to pull out, tie up, and toss out the door of my room. Sometimes it would break, splattering on the hospital floor, leaving me despondent and embarrassed in my bubble, unable even to clean up my own mess. But this toilet seemed as far away now as it had then.

One more step and the metal tree collapsed on top of me, crushing my weakened body, leaving me gasping for air, hyperventilating, scared, and very sad. *How can I be this sick? Will I ever really get outside? Is all this effort worth it? God, I am so tired and weak.* The nurses rushed in and lifted me onto the bed, trying to calm me and restore my breathing to normal.

The hours and days passed, and almost as quickly as the pneumonia had attacked my body, I got well. Dr. Judith Lyding, the doctor who had supervised the treatment protocol that I was undergoing, called me mercurial. During my two-month stay in the hospital, one day I would be ravaged by fever, the next cheerful and full of spunk. She said she never knew what to expect. I was taken off liquid calories and given real meals, more or less. I was even able to order food. The offering was very limited and didn't sound too appetizing, but it didn't really matter. I just liked the idea of solid cuisine. How much pleasure we take in the rituals of life—eating, sitting on a toilet, showering, stepping outside. And we tend to take them for granted until they're taken from us.

One night I was given a menu. The creamed chicken sounded good, so I ordered it. My first solid food!

"Here you are," replied nurse Pat, grinning as she lifted the metal lid of my food dish, knowing how much I was looking forward to eating. It had been almost two months since I had tasted anything but my own vomit.

I stared at my first supper, chagrined. "I can't eat that. It looks like baby vomit."

Pat looked at it, too. "You know, you're right," she commented as she replaced the cover. "We're going out for burritos. Would you like one?"

My eyes glistened. I loved this nurse. "Do you think it would be okay?"

"Why not?" she replied.

Why not, indeed!

Dr. Lyding walked into my room on my second bite. I couldn't taste a thing, my taste buds temporarily destroyed by the chemo, but the burrito looked delicious and that was enough for me. I glanced up at her eyes, which were focused directly on my burrito. Too late to hide it under my pillow. I smiled lamely.

"What are you eating?" she inquired.

My grip tightened around the aluminum foil. *She's not getting this from me no matter what.* "A burrito."

"A burrito! Where did you get it?" she asked, dumbfounded.

"The nurses were ordering takeout at the Mexican place, and I made them get me one. I'm okay. I'm feeling good. I couldn't eat the crap they brought up. It looked awful," I said between bites.

Dr. Lyding chuckled, "If you can keep that from coming out both ends, I guess we'll have to let you out of here."

That night I intended to tape both my mouth and butt shut, if necessary. My stay in the hospital had seemed like an eternity, and although I didn't feel great, I tried to convince myself otherwise. Home. Freedom. I could sleep in a real bed, take a bath, go to the store and pick out foods I wanted to eat, whether I could taste them or not. I could go for walks and to the movies. I could rest my head on my husband's shoulder at night.

Early the next morning Dr. Lyding came into my room, smiling.

"Pack up your things. You're going home."

I practically jumped out of bed. I had been awake for the last three hours, hoping I would hear those words. I gave her a big hug.

"Thank you, Dr. Lyding. Thank you for everything."

"You're not out of the woods yet," she reminded me, not dampening my spirits in the least. "I will need to see you once a week, sooner if you have any problems at all. I want you to take your temperature twice a day. If it goes up, I want to see you. Your immune system is still very compromised, so wear your mask, always in public, for at least a few more weeks. We will leave in the catheter to draw blood and in case you need any more medications. And finally, watch what you eat. No salads, sushi, anything too acidic. Your stomach will be a little fragile for a while."

Even though I knew my prognosis for long-term survival was still undetermined, I had survived the treatment that had the greatest chance of eradicating all the cancer from my system. Funky stomach and all, I felt like I was on the road to wellness.

Still smiling, I called Roger to pick me up. On the way to the apartment, we stopped at the park, the beautiful dreamlike park that I had viewed each morning, noon, and night from my womb-room. It was even more glorious close up. We walked slowly two blocks to the end of the park and back. I held on to Roger for support as I shuffled my weakened body over the soft, sweet-smelling grass, smiling like a Cheshire cat the whole way. I looked up at the wide-open sky, feeling the sun's rays on my face, and tilted my head to better hear the chirping of the birds. I sought out each little flower, smelling its delicious fragrance. I spread my arms open wide, marveling at all the space. And before crumpling, wasted, into the car, I stood at the edge of the park, with the hospital behind me, and raised my clenched fists into the air. Another summit! I was back and so alive, so very alive.

In the following days, I would walk six blocks and then eight. I tried driving once but wasn't ready for the hustle and bustle of downtown San Francisco. Two months I had resided in one room. Occasionally the television or radio had been on, but generally it had been quiet. My mind had been clear of any decisions or distractions. All that had been required of me was to lie there peacefully and get well. The "real" world, the one I had previously known, now slammed me in the face. There was too much going on. There were horns and voices, colors and words, movement, commotion everywhere. Someone cut me off and I almost broad-sided them. I couldn't make a snap decision or move quickly. I eased the car over to the curb and sat there with my head on the steering wheel, overwhelmed. I finally took the keys out of the ignition, locked the car, and walked home.

Did I really live this way before? I wondered. *How did I handle all this disturbing noise?* Billboards and lights and signs bombarded my senses. *No more,* I thought. *I want my space to be quiet. I want the sounds I hear to be natural, refreshing, not harsh.*

Two weeks after I left the hospital, I slipped on my sneakers and walked the four blocks to the entrance gate of the Presidio, the densely forested military base perched high above San Francisco Bay. I could never repay our good friends, Jim and Barbara Willenborg, for lending us the guest quarters in their stately home on Broadway. And I thanked God for this glorious day and for giving me another chance. I couldn't get enough of the warmth of the sun on my shoulders and the crunch of the eucalyptus leaves beneath my feet.

As I entered the Presidio, I thought about the joy of living, and I wondered what my future might hold. "Don't know," I heard myself saying, "nor do I particularly care." I was just thrilled to be alive, to truly be on the path to wellness. I knew, first and foremost, that I would concentrate on my peace of mind. If I didn't want to drive, I wouldn't. If I didn't want to be with certain people, good-bye. Before I got sick, I had felt that I must do everything, go everywhere, not miss anything. Well, I had just missed two months of "things," and it hadn't mattered one iota. I vowed to keep that in mind next time we were invited to do something I didn't find appealing.

I followed the path around the Presidio, savoring each step, each precious moment, unwilling to turn around. I was dragging by the time I reached the apartment and finally dropped, exhausted, onto the bed.

The next day I reported to Dr. Lyding. "I walked around the Presidio."

"You what?" came her incredulous reply.

"I was really tired, but I didn't want to retrace my steps."

"That is an eleven-mile walk," she chuckled, shaking her head. "I guess you're going to be fine."

I smiled, thinking of another time and place. A time when my body was strong as a yak, walking for weeks over steep terrain. A place that was magical. One that instilled in me the knowledge that I could dream while I was awake.

CHAPTER 8

Nepal

A mind that is stretched by a new experience
can never go back to its old dimensions.

Oliver Wendell Holmes

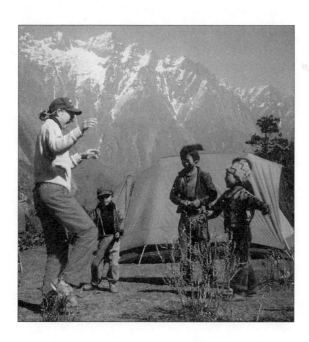

There is a moment of sadness in anticipating the upcoming weeks. The kind of sadness one feels when deep down you realize that things will never be the same. The comfortable security of today's parameters will be replaced by a new way of seeing and thinking and feeling that will shake the old foundation.

———————■———————

The call came on a Thursday afternoon in early January 1989. At the time I was struggling with the creative process, needing to get some designs down on paper for an upcoming deadline. But instead of sketching, I had spent the morning seated at my desk, looking out the window at San Francisco's Union Square, almost catatonic, pencil in hand. *This is not going to be a productive day,* I mused, watching a young couple cross against the light, bringing a Muni bus to a screeching halt. When the phone rang, I welcomed the distraction.

"Laura, this is Lou. I just wanted to let you know that I'm putting together a trek team to join us on the American Kangchenjunga Expedition. Only climbing expeditions were allowed into the area that leads to the Kangchenjunga base camp until a new decision this past fall. Now a select group of trekkers will be able to go into an area that has rarely been seen by Westerners. It will be a unique experience. I figured you might need a challenge. We'd be pleased to have you join us."

"It sounds wonderful, Lou," I heard myself reply. I had listened to many people talk about the Himalayas. The serious climbers had all been there. There was no question that I would love to go to Nepal. "How long, how much, when?" I asked. *Can I leave right now?* crossed my mind.

"You would leave early March and fly into Kathmandu, the capital of Nepal. From there, after a few days of preparation, you would fly to Tapeljung to start your hike in. It will be challenging, about 200 to 250 miles over hilly terrain. My wife, Ingrid, is going to lead the trek to base camp, which will consist of five to ten people plus porters, so you won't have to carry much. It will take about six weeks. We already have a couple of guys with climbing experience from the Seattle area who want to go. There is also a gal from Florida who has signed on. It should be a good group."

I stared at the blank paper in front of me. I had two design assignments due before March. Could I get them finished, along with all the paperwork, before then? Would my clients still be my clients if I took off that much time?

"Send me some information," I replied.

I had already made up my mind. I was going. I couldn't pass up an opportunity like this, to go to Nepal and be a part of a major Himalayan expedition with Lou and many others I knew from Rainier Mountaineering. Kangchenjunga is the third highest mountain in the world, and up until that point no Americans had ever successfully climbed it. What a thrill it would be to take part in what could certainly be a momentous project.

Breaking the news to Roger would not be so easy. My husband and I spent almost all of our time together, becoming more reliant on each other for support and companionship as we moved from town to town—four major moves over the last eighteen years. Other than my travel for work, which was extensive, and my other, shorter, mountain-climbing trips, we had always been together. I knew Roger was not going to be excited about my leaving for six weeks. I formulated in my mind how I was going to approach him. I decided to bring up the subject right away.

"Roger, I need to talk to you," I mentioned that night after dinner.

"What's wrong?" he inquired, concerned.

"Nothing's wrong, I just need to talk to you about something that's come up. Why don't we sit in the living room?"

Roger sat quietly on the sofa, watching me intently as I explained why I had to go on this trek. I told him that I knew I would be gone for a long time and that I loved him and would miss him, but that I also felt this was an opportunity of a lifetime. I detailed why I needed to do this, that I was going to do this, and that I didn't want him to be angry or to try to stop me.

When I finished, he didn't say a word, although it was clear he had been taken aback. I don't know how I would have felt if the tables had been turned, but I could see in his eyes that he was feeling dejected. Six weeks is a long time.

"You didn't even ask if I might want to go," he finally replied.

I looked at Roger. He had never expressed an interest in climbing. Was this something he was really keen on doing, or was he just hurt because he felt I was abandoning him? I knew, ultimately, that this wasn't something Roger wanted to do. I didn't agree with the notion that married people do everything together, even if one of them doesn't really want to.

So on March 28, 1989, I flew alone from San Francisco to Bangkok and on to Kathmandu. As is the case with many major expeditions, a support team of trekkers would follow the climbing team to the mountain, bringing with them mail, extra supplies, and enthusiasm to buoy the summit team. The schedule was for our trek team, led by Ingrid, to arrive several weeks after Lou and his team had established base camp so that we could share in the excitement as the expedition moved up the mountain.

Because of my love of the out-of-doors and my love of adventure, I knew I was embarking on a trip that would very likely influence how I felt about my career and myself and how I would choose to spend my time in the future. I had no idea, however, of the challenges that lay ahead and how emphatically those words would prove to be true.

Kathmandu is a place like no other, startling in its poverty but at the same time exotic and magical with an underlying spirituality that makes up for what the city lacks in cleanliness and creature comforts. An immense temple keeps watch over the town from its vantage point aloft the highest hill in the area. On the main tower are painted Buddha eyes, which stare down every hour of the day, penetrating the souls of all who pass. Dirt streets are lined with side-by-side shacks housing vendors of meat and vegetables for the locals and trinkets for the tourists. An occasional Western-style hotel reflects the increasing number of foreign climbers who pass through Kathmandu on their way to the Himalayas. The lifeblood, flowing through the center of town, is the Trisuli River.

After a day of sightseeing, we stopped to watch a funeral procession make its way through town, halting on the bank of the river. The cremation pyre had already been assembled, the body soon to be incinerated and the ashes scattered in the water.

"Don't they bathe in that river?" questioned John, one of my fellow trekkers.

"Yes, and they wash the vegetables in there, too. So be careful what you eat," replied Ingrid Whittaker. Although we took that warning to heart, half of our trek team spent a long night in the bathroom on or near the toilet.

After several days in the city, we had exhausted our curiosity, bargained for one too many decorative boxes and bracelets, and feared that if we didn't get out in the fresh air of the mountains, we would all get sick. We were elated on day four, when we found out that we were headed for the hills. Elated, that was, until we saw our mode of transportation.

Because of a fuel embargo from India that limited the number of airplanes available to fly, we were to be bused to a small nameless village fifty miles closer to Kathmandu than the originally scheduled airport but an equal distance farther from base camp on Kangchenjunga. The upshot was that our trek in would take several days longer—if we survived the bus ride, which was questionable. We were amazed when we saw the exterior of our vehicle. It was a sight to behold, covered with a collage of florals, street scenes, and religious symbols in brilliant shades of gold and red. Inside was an entirely different matter.

"Watch out for the glass," commented Ingrid, which I noticed about the same time that my eye caught two rusty nails protruding from the sides of the bus. I wasn't aware of the holes in the floor until later, when I watched, mesmerized, as the road passed beneath us. I had given up on sleep, finding it impossible to achieve a comfortable position on the wooden plank that served as my seat and also my bed. For a day and a night we traveled on narrow, unpaved roads, trying to brace ourselves when the driver would get a little too close to the edge, which was bordered only by precipitous dropoffs of a thousand feet or more.

We would hold our breaths and look warily at each other when the driver would stop, frequently on long descents, getting out to fiddle with the brakes under the front of the cab. This happened mostly at night. We had wanted an adventure, and here we were. I was reminded of the axiom, "Be careful what you wish for. You may get it."

Fortunately, we survived the motorized introduction to our journey, and from the first steps of the trek, the bus, all thoughts of Kathmandu, and any concerns at home were left behind. We saw no one for hours, only layers of lush green terracing, fertile with potatoes and rice. Rolling hills on a backdrop of snowcapped mountains bordered a deep, continuous valley that cradled the Ghunza River, which eventually would lead us to the Kangchen-junga base camp, almost two hundred miles away.

Narrow goat paths were pencil-sketched on the steep slopes, meandering up and down thousands of feet in each direction. The faint routes traversed riverbeds and rock slides, barely providing footholds on the steep cliffs that led down to the river. These precarious trails have been dubbed "The Nepalese Highway," since foot travel along this thoroughfare provides the only means of communication between the interior of Nepal and the outside world. It was evident to us early on that we would get all the physical challenge we bargained for and more. That night in camp after a demanding first day, we talked.

"We are out here, totally removed from civilization, without a doctor," one of the guys pointed out.

"The terrain is treacherous. If anyone gets injured, we're on our own," someone else added. "It will be difficult to get someone out of here if they are hurt badly."

"We are going to have to look out for each other," everyone agreed.

My guardian angel came in the form of my tentmate, Sally Chapman, a very pretty, five-foot-seven-inch forty-something blond. Not that I noticed much of that after a day or two. By then I was wearing her extra pair of cotton hiking pants, since I had none (I'd read somewhere that you are supposed to wear skirts while trekking in Nepal), eating her dried fruit, and marveling at her ability to deflect attention away from herself. She was able to make those who came in contact with her feel better than they had before their paths crossed.

A typical exchange would go like this: Someone would ask, "Sally, do you, by any chance, have any extra batteries?"

"Well, of course, I do. Here, these are yours. Thank you for asking," Sally would generously reply.

At night Sally and I would cozy into our small A-frame style tent and reflect on the similarities in our lives. We discussed our athletic endeavors, our mutual fascination with nature, our Native American heritage, and our long marriages, or we would laugh ourselves silly—that is, if we weren't just lying there quietly listening to the Ghunza River. More often than not, we would snuggle into our down-filled bags and let the rush of the water ease our tired bodies and cradle us to sleep. This soothing background sound was less like a lullaby and more like a deep-tissue massage.

The Ghunza is a ferocious river, shaped by steep canyons and forced in torrents around the sides and over the tops of Volkswagen-sized boulders. It roars down from the highest snow-covered peaks in the world, icy cold, descending in swirling rapids and magnificent falls. And it was a bitch to cross.

Makeshift suspension bridges were strung across the river at infrequent intervals, only where it was absolutely necessary. A couple of bamboo poles were often strapped together with twigs, twine, and what looked to be old coat hangers. This conglomeration was then somehow anchored to the riverbanks and made secure. How the engineers of these architectural marvels managed this was baffling. The height of the bridges varied, some swaying precariously as high as sixty feet over the white water below. We came upon one of these high, gravity-defying crossings our first week out.

"You're not serious!" exclaimed one of our most stalwart climbers as his gaze leaped from the bridge down the vast distance to the thundering river. The rest of us were silent, in too much shock to speak. One at a time, however, we proceeded carefully across, keeping our eyes glued to the far bank while we measured our pace so as not to set in motion the makeshift contraption below our feet.

To balance out the discomfort of the bridges came the joy of the villages. "Namaste," the traditional Nepalese greeting, would welcome us in singsong voices from the first children who spotted us. They would stand proudly in their tattered clothes, palms together in front of their faces, prayer style, eyeing us over the tops of their fingers while shy smiles played on their lips. Many of the Nepalese lived in tiny hamlets, in wood and mud huts without running water. There were no schools, no hospitals, not a change of clothing. But they appeared to be some of the happiest, most contented people on the face of the earth. These amiable souls would not beg or steal and were quick with a laugh and a smile. The contrast between their acceptance and joy in so little and our (as Americans) ongoing wish for something bigger and better was striking. There was much to be learned from these gentle people about less being more. The translation of their salutation spoke volumes. One interpretation of *namaste* was: "I honor the place in you in which the entire universe dwells. I honor the place in you which is of love, of truth, of light, and of peace. When you are in that place in you, and I am in that place in me, we are one."

But on the way to our destination, any form of civilization was rare. Mostly we traveled up and down the hillsides seeing no one outside of our group. Day twelve of our trek was an exception—the day we wished the rains would stop. After hours of downpour we were soaked but still moving as fast as we could on the rugged, slippery terrain. Our porters, somewhere behind us, were not yet in sight. The rain turned to hail before we reached a flat, open area and a cave the size of a modest living room. It was already providing shelter for several farmers and a couple of cows. This was to be our campsite as soon as our bags arrived. We huddled in the cave with the current residents for over an hour, sodden and shivering, using one another's body heat to ward off hypothermia. When the tents arrived, they were put up in a hurry, everyone anxious to get out of the cold and into dry clothes.

"I am freezing," I commented as I stripped off my rain jacket, dropping it in the corner of the tent. "So much for the waterproofness of this thing." Next came my long underwear, dripping.

I heard Sally gasp, and I turned to see what was wrong. "Oh my God," she muttered, staring at me. "Leeches. You're covered with leeches. Hold still and I'll pluck them off."

The remaining daylight hours we spent in our tent, mostly naked, searching our own bodies and each other's, pulling off leeches from backs, legs, and arms. Although these bloodsuckers presented no real danger, it was nonetheless unnerving knowing they had somehow slipped into our clothing and onto our bodies and were merrily feasting away.

As in most situations, the crisis passed fairly quickly. The next day dawned crystal clear, the mountains and their blanket of greenery glistening from the previous day's cleansing. Marveling at the fresh beauty around us, we broke camp and were once again under way.

The higher we trekked, the more treacherous the terrain became. En route to Kambachen at 12,000 feet, we had to traverse a long, very steep rock slide. Before we started onto the rock field, a herd of mountain sheep farther up the hill began kicking loose boulders down the slope, nearly onto the heads of our cook and several porters who had already started across the slope. Two of the porters huddled under an overhang while rocks large enough to knock them out thundered down the slope beside them. The cook managed to hustle out of the way in one direction, while another porter ran hurriedly to our location. Eventually the other two made it off the slope amid frantic shouts of "rock," leaving their baskets and supplies behind. It was frightening watching the loose rocks gather speed, barely missing members of our team. One hit would have been a disaster.

After what seemed like an eternity, the rocks came with less regularity, and the remaining porters headed across one at a time with everyone watching the slopes above. When the porters reached the other side safely, we were next. More than forty minutes had already gone by. Ingrid Whittaker was the first of the trekkers to start, and the rocks gave way from above as she was midway across. At first she didn't hear our warning and nearly got blindsided. Finally, she heard our cries and frantically scrambled out of danger.

One by one we ventured forth across the rough slope. When my turn came, I took off as fast as I could, only to feel my footing give out rapidly halfway across. I landed face down, skinning my knee and leg and bruising my hand. Realizing the danger, I got up immediately and hobbled to the boulder overhang, where I caught my breath. My heart was pounding less from the altitude or exertion than from the fear of getting swept away by the falling fragments. What had seemed plenty frightening from the sideline was magnified once I was in the middle of the rock slide with virtually no cover. After we had all managed to cross safely, we looked back at what could have been a grave for any one of us and watched a half a dozen massive boulders come crashing down, seemingly out of nowhere, and ricochet off the landing where we had stood for almost an hour. They literally would have taken us with them.

When we reached base camp at Pang Pema at 16,500 feet two weeks after we had started, Ingrid ran into Lou's outstretched arms. Lou's delight upon seeing our trek team thinly veiled his obvious concern, making even clearer to us the extent of the danger we had been exposed to on this trek. Lou had led his summit team along the same trails, weeks earlier, for the first time. It was more treacherous than he had anticipated, and he had worried about our safety. But, fortunately, we had arrived without mishap. And what a place to be!

Pang Pema sat on a broad plateau that was shadowed by the ominous profile of Kangchenjunga, the five-summited mountain known to the Nepalese as the "Five Treasure Houses of the Snows." Bordering it were the sheer faces of Tent Peak, Nepal Peak, and the Twins. It was impossible not to be overwhelmed by the majesty of nature presenting itself to us after our long walk in. The trip had been well worth it.

But reaching base camp and later climbing up to Camp One was not the culmination of the trek for me. It was just a beginning. For one thing, I found a lifelong friend in Sally Chapman. Lou would often say, "A friend is a gift you give yourself." Sally's friendship is an ongoing reminder of a special period of time that I might have missed if I had told Lou no so many months earlier.

Because of all that I learned in the backcountry of Nepal, I set new priorities. I had long loved the beauty of the mountains and the physical and mental rigors of spending time in them, but I had been a weekend warrior, fitting a climb in here or there, not putting it high on my list. All that changed on Kangchenjunga as I sat on the small portable chair in the cook tent, listening to the climbers higher up on the mountain and talking to those left behind, who were waiting their turn. Some of the most accomplished American mountaineers waited in anticipation for their shot on the upper mountain and eventually the summit. We, the trek team, had reached our intended goal of base camp, and some of us had the opportunity to go to Camp One, but there our climb ended. Feeling the excitement and intensity of the summit climbers, I wanted their experience for myself.

That night I wrote in my diary:

How incredible it is to stand at the base of this formidable mountain. To look up at its peaks beckoning those that have chosen the mountains as a way of life. To look at its quiet, solid masses, at the same time so docile and so dangerous. As I admire its beauty, I imagine the climbers who toil above, ignoring discomfort and pain to stand for one brief moment on the top, to know that in their hearts and souls that for that short period of time (long in preparation), they have accomplished what so few have or are able to. They have confronted nature and for one brief moment have won the challenge. They have pushed beyond their limits for the satisfaction that is rightfully theirs. There is a purity of purpose that attracts me to this sport. I wonder, silently, if one day I will look down from that great height and what it will take to get there.

I also wrote, "I will walk a little taller when I go home, because I'm more comfortable in my shoes." But I had no idea, then, where my shoes would take me.

CHAPTER 9

Intimacy

There is always a thread that leads
back to beginnings and continues
into the uncharted future.

Anonymous

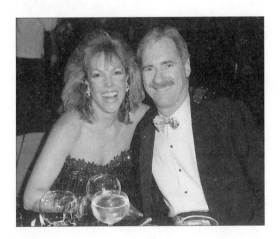

I want to dance again and laugh out loud and howl at the moon. I want to let loose and pretend that life didn't twist and bend and try to break me. I want to pretend that I am invincible once again.

———■———

"You grow 'em, we glow 'em" read a sign in the window of a drugstore on San Francisco's eccentric Polk Street, not far from the Pacific Presbyterian Hospital. It was there that Roger bought the condoms.

"When you have sex again, and you should start as soon as possible," said Dr. Grant, my oncologist, "Roger will have to wear protection. Your immune system is still very vulnerable."

It had been a very long time since Roger and I had even thought about "protection." I had been on the pill for ten years before coming to the conclusion that I didn't want whatever was in those little tablets in my system any longer. After numerous discussions, Roger and I had decided that I would get my tubes tied, thus making all birth control unnecessary. In fact, the last time the concept had entered my mind was when the leading lady in the movie *Skin Deep* had insisted that her lovers wear glow-in-the-dark condoms. I chuckled at the memory.

"If we have to use a condom, then it has to be fun," I informed my husband on the way to Polk Street, making light of our mission. I was nervous. It had been months since we had made love. In the last two months, I had had no human contact at all. Additionally, the intense doses of chemotherapy I had been given had thrown me into early menopause. Would it be painful to have sex? Would I even want to? I knew how important it was for both of us to be close again, to regain the intimacy we'd had before. And I wanted that. So many nights in the hospital I had hugged Gordo to my chest, crying into his fur. I was so lonely. I missed hugs and kisses, a simple touch.

But I didn't feel sexy. My body had been abused by so many drugs, my mind warped by fear and confusion. My mode for the last months had been survival, not pleasure. I wasn't sure I knew how to begin again.

But Roger came out of the store holding a small packet of Day-Glo green rubbers, which helped to ease the tension. Driving back to the house, we chuckled like children breaking the rules.

That first night, with our glow-in-the-dark condom lighting the way, we tried unsuccessfully to make love. It felt wonderful to lie in each other's arms, but our lovemaking didn't go beyond that. I felt as if someone had sewn up my private parts. Sorry, no admittance. Roger and I had always had good sex. In the past, abundant good sex. But now things were different.

"It's so painful when we make love," I told my oncologist at my six-month checkup. "I bleed every time. I hate this. I don't know what to do."

"Get Replens," she said. "It's a vaginal moisturizer."

Whoever invented Replens must have known that breast cancer was on the rise. Not only did the cost of the product start out ungodly expensive, the price kept going up. I used it religiously, regardless, following the instructions on the package and the advice of my doctor. It seemed to help some, but it did not eliminate the fact that I no longer felt attractive.

My breast was chopped up from the lumpectomy, my hair was an inch long, and I was surviving cancer (nine months and counting). Looking or feeling provocative did not seem to be a high priority. Yet I missed our former intimacy, and so did my husband.

"I need to feel close to you. I want us to make love. I'll go real slowly," Roger mentioned from time to time. And we would try, and it would hurt.

One day we discovered Astroglide, which comes in a small plastic bottle, sort of the male counterpart to Replens. Who thinks up these names? We called it Visine because of the similar-looking container and because of a particular incident. One morning just after I had walked into the kitchen to start breakfast, I heard Roger call from near the bedroom, "Laura."

"Yes, dear," I responded as I squinted down the hall. He was waving a small bottle in the air. *Visine? Why is he waving a bottle of eye solution at me*? Roger frequently used Visine in the morning. Of course, what he was waving around wasn't eyedrops.

Visine and Replens aside, it took a long time, with Roger's loving encouragement, to get into sex again, and even years later I couldn't quite envision myself in the black lacy garter belt and push-up bra that I had once worn.

The first year after treatment, sexy underwear was the furthest thing from my mind. I cried almost daily in my confusion and discomfort. I was through with my treatment, my hair had grown back, and I was well. Right? Wrong. Neither physically nor mentally. My mental distress did not lend itself to physical intimacy. At night I would curl up on my side of the bed and leak tears into my pillow. Roger would put a comforting hand on my shoulder, but when I didn't respond he would remove it, sigh, and roll over, knowing he was unable to help me deal with whatever demons were playing havoc with my mind.

Roger continued to be loving and supportive, but even for him my tears got to be too much. "Are you ever going to stop crying?" Roger asked one evening, when there was a brief lull in the flow.

"No, never," I replied, more than halfway believing it.

The tears would come when I least expected them and for no apparent reason. I was confused and frazzled by the responsibilities that were once again part of my life. *I almost died,* I thought. *Can't I just live? Do I really have to think about dinner, weekend plans, money, sex?* At times I would crawl into bed, pull the sheet over my head, and roll up in a ball, back to the womb, refusing to think about anything.

I was so thankful to be out of the hospital, grateful for my newfound freedom, for the hot showers and quiet nights, for Roger's strong arms, which wrapped around me with loving hugs. But I would sit there and cry. I wanted to take myself back in time, before all this happened. I cried for what was lost—for the familiar life, for the old me, the long-haired, blond, wild and crazy me, the one who smiled incessantly and thought life went on forever. The one who looked forward to good, healthy sex. God, it was fun while it lasted.

I didn't understand, then, that I was in the middle of a process, the process required to get through any crisis. I had been inundated with drugs, my life turned upside down. The body and mind required time to heal, to sort things out. Even with all the much-needed hugs and kind words, I would have to work through this slowly, much like I used to climb mountains, one step at a time, listening closely to the rhythms of my mind and body, not rushing things.

"I feel like my life is a puzzle, placed in a box, then shaken up and dumped on the floor for me to put back together. The only problem is the pieces aren't the same, and there are several missing," I told Roger one night. "For the first time in my life, I don't know where to begin." We both knew it would take patience. Long after my hair grew back and I looked healthy again, I would still be adjusting to all that I had been through, still juggling pieces of the puzzle to fill in the gaps.

Because intercourse was uncomfortable, it had become more of a responsibility and less of a pleasure. But I knew, as with the other gaps in my life, that I would have to work on restoring some of the intimacy we had before—for Roger and for me.

I would often seek the comfort of the hills, going for long, solitary walks. I would feel nature's calm soothing me, releasing my anxiety. "Just let things happen," the wind would say. "Not to worry," the trees would whistle. "All things in their own time," the birds would sing.

And all things did work out in time, and before Roger and I knew it, we were having regular sex, perhaps not with the same abandon as before, but with a greater appreciation for each other and for what both of us had been through. We would rebuild our lives together, finding new common ground, a new way to be lovers.

CHAPTER 10

Reentry

The trick is what one emphasizes. We either make ourselves miserable or we make ourselves strong. The amount of effort is the same.

Carlos Castaneda

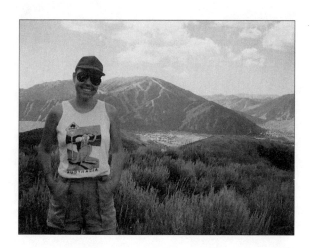

I must look at myself as a person, not as some ideal that, through years of molding, people will look at and marvel. Think, Laura, only of the quiet inner self. What will it take for the calm contentment, easy enjoyment of it all? The nonjudgmental acceptance of my personal being as well as of those around me?

———————■———————

One of my first requests on leaving the hospital—after food, of course, although I still couldn't taste anything—was to see a movie. What I wanted to see was *Pretty Woman,* a choice I regretted almost the minute the movie started. The day of the movie I was wearing my short-cut, practical wig—not that it mattered, since I was bald under all of them. But Julia Roberts not only was not bald, she had this incredible flowing mane of hair that spread everywhere, over her clothes, over the bubbles in the bathtub, over Richard Gere. I wondered if I would ever have long hair again and how many months it might be until I had any hair at all.

Two weeks after I was released from the hospital, my sister-in-law Sandy came out to San Francisco to visit. I would remain in this city for another two months undergoing radiation, the last of my medical treatments. When Sandy arrived our first stop was Nordstrom, because I was looking for a cocktail dress for the upcoming hospital ball in Sun Valley. Roger and I had attended this annual event last December, the day after my initial appointment with Dr. Campanale and two days before my hastily scheduled biopsy. I wanted my doctors at home to know I was back, that I was going to be okay.

Sandy and I headed straight for the evening department, and I quickly spotted the perfect dress. I pulled it from the rack and headed to the nearest dressing room. I surfaced several minutes later.

"You look ridiculous," observed Sandy as I stepped out from behind the door of the changing room.

I looked down at the expanse of black and white sequins, disappointed. I liked this dress a lot, and besides, I didn't feel like trying on more than one. "Why don't you like it?" I asked.

"I like the dress, especially with the face mask," she giggled in reply. "But why didn't you take off your jeans, and where's your hair?"

"It was too much trouble to take off my jeans, and my wig kept getting caught in the sequins. I don't have a lot of energy," I replied, glancing around the clothing racks, wondering who else might be amused by my plight. I noticed two Nordstrom employees discreetly looking the other way. When I checked my image in the mirror, I had to chuckle. Indeed, I looked like a mannequin in midchange, going from sportswear to cocktail, the phantom window dresser interrupted by a phone call, not quite able to complete the transformation. I bought the dress. I knew it would always bring a smile to my face.

Back in the apartment, I was exhausted. Even though I walked daily, two months in a hospital bed had taken its toll. I hung up my new dress and set my wig on the dresser. Sitting on the bed, I rubbed the muscles in my neck. I was still trying to work out the stiffness and various aches and pains caused by so many endless hours of lying in one position. The chest catheter, which fortunately had been removed two weeks after my release, hadn't allowed for much freedom of movement. With the catheter on my right side and the surgery on my left, I had mostly slept flat on my back.

I flexed my legs, feeling for any muscle tone, not finding much. But I was thankful that the arthritis was gone. After the final chemo treatment, I was slowly weaned off of the steroids. Miraculously, my joints began to function again and I could move around without the previous discomfort.

I raised my arm over my head and squeezed my fist several times. I was spending three days a week at the lymphedema clinic trying to lessen the swelling in my arm, a result of removing my underarm lymph nodes. It seemed to be working.

The seven weeks of radiation therapy—"just in case," the doctors said—slipped by quickly. After the bone marrow treatment in the hospital, there was no sign of cancer in my body, but radiation would help ensure that it didn't resurface. Each morning, five days a week, I would walk the mile to the hospital, then after treatment the mile home, stopping in every park along the way and window-shopping in between.

On July 11, 1990, Roger and I headed home to Idaho. I know I glowed. Not only was I alive, out of the hospital, finished with treatment, but I was headed back to Sun Valley. On our final night in the Bay Area, we joined close friends of ours at their house for dinner. Their young son knew I had been in the hospital, and I smiled to myself remembering the question he had asked his mom, "Did Mrs. Evans get a face-lift?" *Not a face-lift, dear boy, a life-lift.* As Roger and I drove through Nevada, another wave of intense feelings washed over me. I was going home. My stomach churned with butterflies, and tears flowed freely from my eyes. Home. My friends. The mountains. There had been moments when I wasn't sure if I would be making this return trip. I believed deep down that I would leave San Francisco, but at times it felt like the treatments would go on forever, never allowing me a life of my own.

Blessedly, on July 12 we were back in our beloved Wood River Valley, just in time for one of the big events of the summer. Anxious to see many of our friends and to celebrate my return, we dressed up in our lightweight summer finery and headed to Bellevue for the annual polo matches.

Bouquets of brilliant balloons festively lined the tents, each balloon containing a small slip of paper on which was written the name of a surprise gift. Colorful ornaments and decorations danced gaily in the breeze.

The sun, high overhead, made the crystal glasses glisten. Bright light glowed off the expanse of green playing field and twinkled off the polo mallets. Soft voices mingled with the pounding of hooves and the lighthearted laughter that drifted throughout, surrounding me in a warm embrace.

I smiled, appreciating all my friends, this glorious day. I felt feminine, if not quite sexy, in my backless party dress. I had bought it in San Francisco shortly after purchasing the sequined number, with the protective mask still over my nose and mouth. I couldn't resist all the beautiful roses in the chintz fabric.

I had been back home in Sun Valley for a week, and this was my first outing sans mask. God, it felt good to be alive.

I peered out from under my stylish, oversized black straw hat and laughed inwardly. Some of these people didn't know that under my hat was nothing but a shiny, smooth noggin.

Bald is not beautiful, I had decided. It was, most assuredly, unnatural. But right now, in this place and time, I was just happy to be alive, and it didn't matter that I was bald.

I took my husband's hand. "Roger, I want a balloon. Will you buy me a balloon? A special prize to celebrate my homecoming."

"Sure, sweetie," he responded as I led him in the direction of the main tent.

"Which color?" he asked, looking up at a rainbow selection.

"Red, my favorite," I replied instantly.

He handed me a red balloon and I quickly popped it, smiling in anticipation. But as I read the small slip of paper that described my surprise gift, the grin froze on my face.

"What's wrong?" asked my suddenly concerned husband.

"I don't believe this," I said.

"What?" he asked again.

"I won a haircut!"

■ ■ ■

Roger and I took our first vacation together six months after I completed my treatment. We were going to Mexico with our good buddy, Ted Dale. Ted had a place on the beach in Baja. Miles of soft sand lay two steps from the back door of his *casita*. It sounded glorious. We spent days in preparation, like little kids, pulling out all our summer clothes, bathing suits, shorts, T-shirts, snorkels, and fins, spreading them out on the bed, giddy in anticipation of our upcoming holiday.

Roger and Ted had worked together since the early seventies, first in commercial real estate and later in partnership on various real estate developments. Over the years we had all become close friends.

Less than a year before our scheduled trip, I remember telling Ted at his Christmas party about my cancer diagnosis.

"That is the worst thing I have ever heard," he replied.

"The worst?" I asked. "Ever?"

"Yes," he replied.

Even though Ted was prone to exaggeration, I knew he was sincere in his concern. But that diagnosis was behind us. We were headed to Mexico. The worst was over. Nothing would spoil our vacation. Unless I did the unthinkable and left my luggage at home.

It was still dark when we loaded up the car for the three-hour drive to Boise, where we would catch a 9:30 A.M. flight to

San Jose del Cabo. It wasn't until we were standing in front of the airline counter that I realized, with abject horror, that we only had two bags, not three, and that the one missing was mine. How could this be? Our first special trip and I had nothing to wear, no swimsuit, no shorts, none of the things I had so carefully selected and laid out.

One of the unpleasant and unanticipated side effects of chemotherapy is memory loss. It affects people to varying degrees, and memory returns partially, in installments, if you're lucky. Because of the extreme doses I had been given, I was now borderline Alzheimer. I have learned the hard way to make lists whenever anything comes to mind and to recheck everything—luggage, location of glasses, keys, and so forth.

Fortunately, the Mexico trip was saved through the kindness of our part-time cleaning woman, who retrieved my suitcase from our bedroom, where it sat abandoned, and ferried it to the airport for the next flight out.

North of Cabo San Lucas, a short walk from the Hotel Palmilla, is a gated complex of four two-story, whitewashed homes, shoulder to shoulder around a circular drive, contrasting starkly with the surrounding desert. Abundant bougainvillea plants and flowering cacti line the cul-de-sac. We pulled up in front of the first house on the right.

"This is ours, the one with the fountain that has never worked," motioned Ted, pulling luggage from the trunk of the car.

The front door was a massive plank of mesquite wood. It opened onto a vast expanse of Mexican tile that filled the upstairs landing, then wound down a circular staircase to a wall of sliding glass. Through these windows we could view the ocean, spread out before us like an open clam, delicious and inviting. One of the first things I had noticed when I was released from the hospital is how big everything looked. After my two-month confinement in a closet-sized chamber, everything seemed spacious:

hallways, bathrooms, bedrooms. But Ted's hideaway was, without discussion, grand. I was suddenly transported a million miles from the hospital and from the discomfort, pain, and confusion of the last eleven months. *This is good*, I thought as I looked around. *Better than good.*

The plans for the next day were to go swimming, walk on the beach, and fish for tuna in order to stock our *cocina* for the week. I love fresh fish, especially Ahi tuna.

But I don't necessarily love the process of fishing. Unaware until the following morning that I was delegated to the fishing patrol, I rose reluctantly at 5:00 A.M. *Do the fish really know what time of day it is?* I thought. *Can't we do this in a few hours, when civilized people get up?*

Half awake, Roger and I walked slowly, carefully down the beach, avoiding the dark outlines that were no doubt the rocks we had seen from the deck the night before. Ahead, we could see the faint light of the fishing shack. It was there we would find out which ponga boat and boatmaster were ours. I don't fish much, and I don't know what I expected in terms of a fishing boat, but certainly more than a wooden dinghy. We climbed into the small boat gingerly, and with our two mute, Mexican guides we sped out to sea.

I consider myself normal, at least in terms of my constitution. When I wake up in the morning at a reasonable hour, I have to go to the bathroom, and not just to pee. This fact crossed my mind as we headed out farther and farther, seemingly to the Caribbean. We had been motoring for hours with no sign of letting up. My body was suddenly wide awake, ready to begin the day's routine.

"Roger, I have to go to the bathroom, soon," I whispered, glancing at the two Mexicans who had been spit-polishing this weathered vessel, their pride and joy, ever since we left port.

"There isn't a bathroom on board," he replied.

"No kidding. I have to go, nonetheless. Now! I can't hold it," I stated as I glanced uncomfortably at our escorts. "I can't go in their boat."

"Hang it over the side," Roger casually commented.

"I can't hang it over the side. I have to poop," I explained, exasperated.

Moments later, I was in the middle of the Sea of Cortez, struggling to get my shorts off before it was too late. I refused to be embarrassed. *This is perfectly natural,* I told myself. *We all go to the bathroom.* As I was treading water trying to get back into my shorts, I came face-to-face with a large floating object. "Oh, no," I muttered as I yanked up my shorts and started to swim away as fast as I could. *Oh, God,* I thought as I glanced over my shoulder.

"Laura, where are you going?" asked Roger in wonderment.

I ignored him and swam harder, farther from my excrement, which appeared to be following me, and farther from the boat. Six months earlier I had been in a sterile room, my immune system at risk, and now I was in the middle of the ocean being chased by a giant turd.

"Ooh la la, *marlino,*" sang the captain, laughing and pointing in my direction. This from the boatman who had not spoken a word for the entire three hours since our departure. *Very funny. Ha, ha.*

That night, back in our *casita,* the morning's embarrassment was eased by the wonderful-tasting tuna and the knowledge that two days hence I would be back home and would probably never see this comedian of a captain again.

■ ■ ■

The week we returned to Sun Valley I started hiking again, easing into it. My first outing was up the service road on Dollar Mountain, eight hundred vertical feet spread out over three-quarters of a mile. My heart was pumping when I reached the top, both from the exertion and the exhilaration of being back in my boots. From the top of Dollar, I could see the entire Wood River Valley stretching from Elkhorn through Ketchum to Warm Springs. It felt so good to be on a summit again, however small.

From my vantage point, I could also see the surrounding peaks, all of them rising above where I stood. And I knew that was where I wanted to be.

After two more trips up Dollar, I hiked Proctor Mountain, four hundred feet higher. As I wound through the aspens, I looked down at where I had been a week earlier and smiled. My legs felt strong and my heart soared. I was back in the mountains that I loved. I felt healthy and alive, and little by little the mantle of sadness slipped away. The worst was behind me. I had been sick, but now I was getting well.

I supplemented hiking with aerobic workouts, weight training, and, in the winter, skiing. Gradually my muscle tone increased. Through hours of walking my hand up a wall, I was able to break down the scar tissue from my operation and regain full range of motion of my arm. The swelling from the lymphedema melted completely away. Yoga and massage relaxed my crimped back and sides, and finally in the spring, a year after my release, I was ready for Baldy. Nine o' clock that morning, I put on two pairs of hiking socks and slipped an extra bottle of water into my fanny pack. It was seventy degrees without a cloud in the sky. This would be a big challenge, 3,300 feet of vertical, but I had all day, and I intended to use every bit of it if necessary.

Heading up the trail, I smiled to myself and to the squirrels that would occasionally scamper by and to the trees that waved at me as I passed and to the few flowers that tenaciously clung to the rocky hillsides. I thought about how often I had looked but not really noticed the beauty that surrounded me. Every leaf and twig seemed more alive, more vibrant. I tested my battered lungs with five or six pressure breaths. Fill up the lungs, purse the lips, blow. My poor lungs. I had gotten pneumonia three times in the past year, but now my lungs responded, forcing the air out between my teeth.

I slowed down my pace so I could go for an hour without stopping and decreased my effort by rest stepping, moving one foot at a time, relaxing my body weight on my locked back leg. Three and a half hours after I started, I willed myself up the final few feet to the Lookout Lodge, perched atop Baldy's Challenger lift. I looked down at the valley floor, thousands of feet below me. I had come a long way. My body had not let me down after all. I allowed myself the thought that perhaps I would climb again.

That night I thought about Kilimanjaro, about the trip I'd had to cancel when I got the cancer diagnosis. I thought about a dream that was unfulfilled.

CHAPTER 11

Kilimanjaro

We're given second chances every day
of our lives. We don't usually take them,
but they're there for the taking.

Andrew M. Greeley

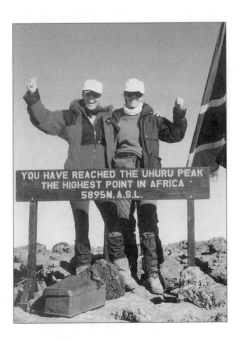

In two weeks, I leave for Africa. A long-awaited dream, but I am ambivalent. Certainly, I am excited. Perhaps all the training, that almost singular focus, has tempered my enthusiasm. Today I climbed Baldy for the fortieth time this summer, 3,300 vertical feet. My total must be around 130,000 feet. I think I can manage a 19,000-foot peak, but I just want to get on with it. I have waited so long, what feels like a lifetime.

———————■———————

It had been six years since I first visited Africa. Africa had been one of the destinations on an around-the-world trip my husband and I took in 1986, compliments of my frequent flyer miles.

"It will be difficult to take off three months," my husband had responded to my suggestion that we cash in the miles I had earned from all my travel.

"We can't not do this," I retorted. "We have two free first-class tickets around the world. We have to use them. We'll kick ourselves forever if we don't take advantage of this opportunity."

We decided to go for it and spent a delightful year planning the trip. It was one of the most fun years of our life together, researching all the places we'd ever dreamed of visiting: Greece, Egypt, Kenya, Thailand, Bali, Australia, New Zealand, Fiji. Then we spent three glorious months traveling to all of them.

But that had been six years ago. It felt more like twenty. Once again I was headed back to Africa, this time for some unfinished business: to climb Kilimanjaro.

Two weeks of packing and last-minute details slipped quickly by, and I was on my way. When I landed in Nairobi, the capital of Kenya, everything seemed different—busier and dirtier than I had remembered. But of course I didn't want to be in Nairobi. I wanted to be in the mountains. And besides, my memory was suspect. Of course, everyone's memory departs from reality; that's why we all have different recollections, sometimes very different interpretations, of the same event. But the sad fact for me was that I really didn't remember. The drugs, and maybe the whole trauma of what I had been through with cancer, left gaps in my memory. This had come to light more than any other time in the Florida home of Sally Chapman, six months before I departed for Africa.

"This is my favorite thing in the whole world," Sally had told me, sitting cross-legged on the wooden floor of her living room. I watched as she placed an antique Tibetan drum gently on the floor in front of her, picking up the piece of notepaper that accompanied it. I wondered why this was so special and why it was so important for her to point it out to me.

She began to unfold and read the paper: "Sally, I think you once told me that the gifts that mean the most to give are the ones that mean the most to the giver. This is a special remembrance of a very special time and place that I will long remember. It has now found its rightful home. Merry Christmas. Love, Laura."

Looking over at the paper in Sally's hands, I recognized the handwriting moments before I recognized the words. I had written this. I had given this gift to Sally, debating because I liked it so much, knowing she would like it more. And I had totally forgotten.

What else have I forgotten? I wondered, wandering the streets of Nairobi. *I know I've forgotten who I am, or I just don't know anymore. Maybe this climb will help sort things out.*

The trip, planned and led by Peter and Erika Whittaker of Summits Adventure Travel, started with a safari. Our outpost was

Paradise Camp in the Masai Mara region of Kenya, geographically an extension of Tanzania's world-famous Serengeti National Park. Aptly named, Paradise consisted of a dozen or so deluxe tents nestled in a wooded area stretched along the Mara River. Each tent was set up on a cement floor and divided into two rooms. The front room was covered with a rattan rug and housed two twin beds with elephant-printed spreads, a small wooden writing desk and chair, and a collapsible suitcase rack. Lanterns lit the room, and flashlights were within easy reach for any night excursions. The back room was the toilet and shower. Two oversized canvas bags hung from its ceiling and were filled each morning with boiling water by the natives who maintained the camp. The accommodations were perfectly designed to give one the feeling that here, in this remote part of the world, time was standing still. It could just as easily have been 1942 as 1992.

Our neighbors were of the four-legged variety: hippos, who kept pretty much to the water, thank God; elephants, who more often than not would wreak havoc in the campground, barreling through tents before our porters could ward them off; and baboons, the most gregarious of them all. One particularly dashing member of this species perched himself on a rock near the entrance to the camp. Here he sat, day and night, for as long as we were there, brandishing an erection that he seemed to be particularly proud of. I think he even winked at a couple of my team members.

Our group consisted mostly of women, young women who were friends of my sister Lisa. I had asked both of my sisters to join me. "This will be a great way for us to spend time together, getting in shape, far away from kids, work, obligations. And what a great adventure," I had tried to convince them both.

"I'd love to," Martha, my middle sister, had replied. "I've always wanted to go to Africa and I'd love to go with you, but I don't know if I can convince my husband. He works so hard.

Who will take care of all the kids? And is it dangerous? I've never climbed before. What if something happened to me? I can't leave David with five kids."

"I'm going," my youngest sister, Lisa, said without hesitation. "I can get into shape by then. Mike can take care of the kids. I deserve this. I have some friends who will probably want to go, too. Is that okay?"

"Yes, Liz."

Lisa is the last of the litter, the baby, seven years younger than I. She has an irrepressible naïveté that is disarming. Even with four kids of her own, she has a childlike quality. You can never be sure what will come out of her mouth. As we safaried through the African game preserves, it was a challenge for Lisa to contain her exuberance and not scare off the animals.

The last night in camp, the Masai danced. No one spoke as the natives, clad only in draped red loincloths and carrying their hunting spears, circled around us in the darkness. There were twenty of them, each with his own distinctive chant. The rhythmic sounds of their breathing, air forced deep from the stomach, grew louder as they circled faster and faster. The continuous movement and the mesmerizing sound of their mantras held us in a web, unable to move and only barely able to breathe. Was it like this for the animals who succumbed to the bravery of Masai hunting on foot, with only spears?

That night I thought about the climb, only a few days away. I knew that it would take this kind of concentration, the warrior's ability to focus inward and summon up every ounce of energy, forcing the energy, to maintain the stamina and strength needed to reach my goal, the summit of Kilimanjaro. Although I had successfully climbed Mount Rainier three months before this trip, my chemo-battered lungs were untested at higher altitudes. As I watched the dancers, I thought, *No matter how difficult the climb might become, I will stay mentally strong. I will hold a visualization of me standing on the top of this peak firmly etched in my brain.*

Kilimanjaro, for me and for many others, has an almost mystical quality. This dormant volcano, situated in Tanzania near the border of Kenya, came into being some two million years ago. Some say its name means "Shining Mountain" or "Mountain of Greatness." But the name may have been derived from a local word, *Kilemieiroya,* meaning "the mountain cannot be conquered." At over 19,000 feet, it is the highest mountain in Africa and therefore is one of the seven continental summits. It presented a very real challenge.

Two days after the thrilling Masai dance we started our climb, taking the less traveled Machame route up the back side. I had been restless for a couple of nights prior to our departure, eager to get going, eager to test my mettle. My disgruntled attitude changed the minute we started hiking. As usual, my mood brightened once we started moving toward our goal.

Patience is not one of my virtues. In fact, it is one of my life-long lessons. Part of the reason I climb is because it requires perseverance. In the mountains, you can go only so fast without getting sick. You have to go at a comfortable, measured rate. I find a great deal of wisdom in Emerson's reflection, "Adopt the pace of nature: her secret is patience."

Once we were under way, I was mellow, enjoying the exotic beauty of the thick undergrowth that all but swallowed up the narrow trail we traveled. A jungle of hanging moss draped above our heads eerily outlined the route. Five miles into it, we reached Camp One at an elevation of 9,850 feet. Other than two metal shacks, partially hidden in the trees where the porters would reside, and areas of flattened vegetation, we saw no evidence of civilization.

The porters spread out the gear, and we went to work setting up camp. Lisa and I found a level, grassy area twenty feet down from the "common area" where we would cook and eat. As we unloaded our duffels, I could tell Lisa was nervous about the days that lay ahead.

"How come we're so different? How do you just keep going? I get tired and I want to just sit down. It's so hard," Lisa confessed.

I looked at my baby sister. She was as tough as they come but sometimes had lapses in willpower. "You have to want it, Liz. You have to really want it. Don't think about being tired or what hurts. Think only about the summit and how much you want to stand up there with me. If you want it enough, you can do it."

She nodded agreement but didn't seem totally convinced.

"Someone once told me," I continued, "that if you don't invest very much, then defeat doesn't hurt very much and winning isn't very exciting. Something to think about."

It didn't help that Lisa got diarrhea, as did we all. But she seemed to be the worst hit. That first night she was up thirteen times, weeding her way through the forest to the trench that was our latrine. Neither of us got much sleep that night, but when we broke camp the following morning, we were ready for a new day.

For close to seven hours we hiked up and across the Shira Plateau. It was shorts and T-shirt weather, but a veil of haze kept it from being too hot. We rose gradually with the terrain, one climber after another, following a well-defined track. The lower rain forests, which had enveloped us the day before, dissolved in mists of fog that shrouded barren rock formations. The moonscape terrain offered up none of the advertised wild eland, a type of antelope, but we were afforded our first glimpse of the glaciers on Kilimanjaro.

We stopped for lunch and stared at the massive, glistening, and slightly intimidating flanks of our intended goal.

"Is this the route we take?" one of the women wanted to know.

"Actually, no," Peter answered. "We traverse around the glacier, up through a fairly steep part, then straight up to the summit. We will be on very little snow and ice."

There were several sighs of relief. We had understood that Kilimanjaro was basically a long trek—up to 19,340 feet. None of us was really prepared to scale an ice wall.

By that afternoon almost everyone was stricken with Montezuma's revenge. Our stomachs would cramp up in protest, forcing us to stop frequently in the shrubs or rocks alongside the route. Dehydration became an issue, and there was legitimate concern as to the health of several of the team members. But we powered down liters of water and started taking Cipro, one of the best antibiotics for the runs.

That night we camped at 12,500 feet. The winds picked up and the temperature dropped. We burrowed into down-filled jackets and huddled within the circle of tents we had arranged among the rocks. Peter built a bonfire, and we watched the big golden orb of a moon as it faded in and out of the clouds, silhouetted against a backdrop of red. We then curled up in our tents and read until even with our headlamps it was too dark to see.

Before we went to sleep Lisa mentioned, "It would be so easy to quit." But she quickly added, "I'm going to make it to the summit."

I thought before I dropped off that it was best not to assume anything. I needed this climb in order to feel, rightly or wrongly, that I was well again. I had trained hard and believed I would make it, but time would tell. I just hoped Lisa would stop even mentioning quitting. Her body might hear that and think it was a good idea.

The following day we stopped every hour to refuel and defuel. We chugged as much water as we could hold and prayed that the Cipro would do its magic. As it was, we ended up using every last bit of toilet paper. We eventually resorted to lemon-scented baby wipes, our tender butts puckering in protest.

On day three I relaxed into the easy pace that Peter had set and let my mind wander. Climbing was an escape for me, removing me from the stresses of everyday life, which at the moment were great.

My working life was a shambles. I had stacks of bills I was struggling to pay, and my career was stalled. A big part of the problem was that I wasn't at all certain that I wanted to keep designing. The incessant travel, the juggling of different clients, trying to be creative when I had so much detail work to tend to—it all took its toll on me. Consequently I had done little since my release from the hospital to drum up work. I wanted a change, a new career. I knew it would all work out eventually, but in my own, predictably human, way, I felt I needed all the answers instantly.

I finally reprimanded myself for not living in the moment and concentrated on the beauty around me. The stark outcroppings of rock, which often appeared to have been dropped randomly from the sky, were soon replaced with towering groundsels or cactus. *What an unusual and interesting climb,* I thought. Every day brought the surprise of a new landscape.

Before long we arrived at the thirty-foot plateau that was Baranco Camp. At 13,000 feet, it butted up against the glacier on one side and dropped off into a steep ravine on the other. Like a mini-oasis, it was surrounded by ten- to twenty-foot cacti, the last of the vegetation on the mountain. From here on up, the trail got steeper. I could just make out where previous climbers had scrambled their way up the rock face. A flat rock for a foot, a large overhang for a hand.

That night as I listened to the quiet of our new surroundings, I heard one of our team members throwing up. He wouldn't admit it yet, but I knew his climb was over. He had been coughing since the second day, and it was becoming clear that he was in the early throes of altitude sickness. This is particularly common on Kilimanjaro. The fairly easy approach leads people to think that they can go up faster, and sometimes farther, than they should. Suddenly they're at 14,000 feet, and they hit the wall. Once altitude sickness strikes, it's merciless and, if unheeded, potentially deadly.

We reached the Barafu Hut at 15,500 feet on day four after a strenuous day of steep, rock-strewn terrain. Our last camp provided minimal flat areas, forcing us to perch our tents wherever we could. As we secured the stakes with rocks, holding the tent and presumably us in place for the night, I looked out at the vast horizon below us. We were but a short distance from the highest point on the continent, and from that vantage point, it was as if we could see forever.

"I'm feeling good," Lisa informed me as we worked. "I'm going to make it!"

"Yes, you are, Liz, and I'm really proud of you," I smiled at her. "Your first climb." I could tell she was empowered by the four days and six thousand vertical feet behind her. But then, like me, she could be very determined.

It was hard to believe that in only six or seven more hours we would be on top. It had been quite a journey—one that I knew wouldn't end with the summit. There were still so many unanswered questions in my mind. I could never forget what I had been through. Death would always be there, lurking behind my every action, daring me to join in the dance. Since I didn't know clearly why I got cancer or if I was, in fact, cured, everything could appear dangerous to my health. I laughed at the irony of climbing; in a way it was one of the least hazardous things I did. At least mentally.

That night I noted in my diary,

Tomorrow I will stand on the long-awaited summit of Kilimanjaro. It has been a long trip, including these last ten days. I'm still trying to find myself, trying to feel secure in who I am now. There are times when I long for the old me. My friends say I look the same, am the same old me, but I'm not. That person is gone forever. Will the new Laura please stand up? Maybe this summit will guide the way.

As I put away pen and paper, I reflected on my favorite Swahili expression, *acuna matata*. It means "no problem." *Acuna matata, acuna matata,* I repeated as if counting sheep. I let the rhythm of the words lull me to sleep. Tomorrow would be a new day. No problem.

We were up again at 1:00 A.M., only a few hours after we had turned in, stumbling around in the dark, making sure our water bottles were full, our sunglasses and sunscreen handy, a snack in our pockets. We bundled up against the cold and sleepily began our final approach to Uhuru Peak.

Slowly, ever so slowly, feeling came back to my fingers and the sky brightened with the promise of a clear day. The early morning sun glanced off the crater rim, twenty feet above. I wiped a tear from the corner of my eye and blew out a couple of breaths.

This is no time to get emotional, Laura. Breathe, I instructed myself.

I looked up again and thought about the day I had left the hospital. Those four tedious, uncomfortable blocks, my lungs burning in an effort to keep up. I saw in my mind's eye the postcard tacked to the bulletin board in my office, a shot of Kilimanjaro, sent two years ago from Peter and the crew on the trip I had helped plan but couldn't attend.

Suddenly I was there. Up ahead was my long-awaited destination, the "Roof of Africa," minutes away. Peter was outlined in front of me in the haze of the early morning light.

"I can't wait, Peter. I know this is obnoxious," I exclaimed as I trotted past him, "but I have to run to the summit."

Breathless, I reached the top, punching my clenched fists skyward, Rocky-style, exulting in my victory. This was my victory over cancer, lymphedema, chemotherapy, drug-induced arthritis, and the odds that were stacked against me. It was a victory that I knew, somewhere deep in my soul, would help me sort out my misgivings and point me in the right direction.

Lisa joined me minutes later, sharing my jubilation. We stood side by side, higher than we had ever been, light-years from the hospital. I hugged my little sister and once again thanked the powers that be for this glorious moment.

"Thank you, Lord," I whispered. "Somehow I'll pay you back."

———■———

CHAPTER 12

Building Bridges

The great thing in the world is not so much where we stand as in what direction we are moving.

Oliver Wendell Holmes

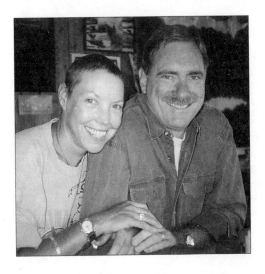

Time has a way of burying insecurities and fears, trying to disguise them with a veneer of wisdom that supposedly comes with age. But they don't go away unless one digs them up, exposes them fully, and then kicks them squarely in the butt out of the house. Exactly what I intend to do with any insecurities, fears, or related actions or thoughts that have brought me to the doorstep of life and death.

———■———

Bonnie Raitt has long been one of my favorite singers. In one of her songs, the lyrics go something like this: "Life is more precious when there is less of it to lose." Since I was diagnosed with breast cancer, I have spent long hours on the phone and in person talking with other women who have had to deal with this life-threatening illness. Without exception, once these people have progressed through the terror and confusion and have come to accept their certain mortality, they have come out the other side with a deep appreciation for life, for the process of living. It seems to be the general consensus among survivors that, yes, every adversity does bear a gift, and for us it is the ability to slow down and smell the roses. For women, in particular, I find that the universe has to drop an anvil on our heads for us to realize that "the time you enjoy wasting is not wasted time."

When I left the hospital, I remember saying, "The sky is bluer, the grass greener, the song of the birds sweeter." I now see the beauty in things that I once would have passed by, and that beauty is magnified tenfold. There is always the lingering thought that it could once again be taken from me, perhaps forever. I now fully understand Emily Dickinson when she said, "To live is so startling, it leaves little time for anything else." I wanted to share my newfound appreciation with others and, hopefully, speed up the painful, emotional process of going through breast cancer. I also wanted to help prepare those who weren't going to survive to deal with the terrifying reality of dying. One needs to prepare for death, not fear it.

In the fall of 1990, with the support and guidance of the Wood River Hospice, I became the volunteer leader of the first wellness group in central Idaho. I clearly recalled the weeks between my initial diagnosis and surgery, when I had realized how much I wanted to talk with other women who had been through what I was about to experience. So many questions I had wanted to ask: "What can I expect? What should I do? What are my options? How will I feel?" There had been no organized support group in the Sun Valley area, and perhaps because of that lack I had found only two women who would talk to me about what they had experienced.

Our first wellness group meetings brought out more women than I ever could have imagined. Most had been through surgery and were either undergoing or had recently finished chemotherapy and/or radiation. The common questions were, "Where do I go from here? How do I get on with my life?"

Doctors, for the most part, are reluctant to counsel their patients on what to eat or drink, when to start an exercise program, and how to contend with early menopause and an emotional system that seems to have run amok. And reading doesn't necessarily help. Every new theory spawns disagreement, and around the corner is always someone else with an even newer idea of how to get healthy. In our wellness group, we gathered up all the information we could find and then discussed it, educating ourselves in the process. This allowed each person to make the decisions she felt worked best for her. We shared our deepest fears, our insecurities, our pain. We became a team, fortified by receptive minds, open ears, and many hugs. Each of us had an ample supply of "good for one free hug" coupons, which we generously distributed. We learned how to nurture ourselves and one another. When a member of our group died, we all mourned, feeling the loss as our own. Studies indicate that people who attend support groups live longer. You have a team, a reason to stay alive. It becomes easier to cope with once-insurmountable obstacles when you face them with fifteen others who have the same or worse problems.

Once Bernie Siegel, before a lecture, instructed all of us in the audience to stand up and talk to at least three people we didn't know to find out why they were there. Of course, all had been seriously ill or lost loved ones and had suffered all manner of trauma, crisis, and disappointment. By the time we sat down, each of us felt we were the lucky one. Longfellow once wrote, "If we could read the secret history of our enemies, we should find in each man's life sorrow and suffering enough to disarm all hostility." It is best to remember that we are not alone.

It is also important to monitor our thoughts. How many of us are fully aware of what notions rattle around in our heads, perhaps hiding in a corner, festering? How many of us have entertained the notion that all our problems would be resolved if we could somehow disappear or if someone else would disappear? My friend Puan, a native of India, once asked me, "How come most Americans allow people to camp out in their heads and shit there?"

How many times do we stew long after the fact over something we said or someone else did? My husband will be driving, and someone else will cut us off.

"Did you see that? What an idiot! I can't believe he did that," Roger will sometimes fume for miles.

"Are you somehow getting back at him with long-distance telepathy?" I wonder aloud. "It doesn't matter. Let it go."

But letting go of our own internal dialogue is even tougher. Many of us berate ourselves inwardly: "I can't believe you said that. I can't believe you did that. You're sure fucked up. You are so stupid. You're a bad person, bad, bad, bad. . . ."

Which reminds me of a great T-shirt. On the front is a sweet but forlorn-looking dog. The caption reads, "My name is No, No, Bad Dog. What's yours?"

Charles Darwin very astutely pointed out, "The highest possible stage in moral culture is when we recognize that we ought to control our thoughts."

I once took a mind study class on relationships during which the discussion turned to jealousy. We've all been there to varying degrees. Our instructor offered one way of dealing with it.

"Okay, your husband or wife—this exercise works both ways, but for the time being we'll say husband—is fooling around. You don't know for sure, but you think maybe he is. Okay, what does she look like? Get a mental picture. Five-foot-nine, long blond hair, big huge breasts in a poor-boy sweater two sizes too small, blue eyes, long red fingernails, short, tight, black leather skirt, four-inch stiletto heels. . . ." By the time you're done, it becomes a joke. You're sitting around eating yourself up over a cartoon character. Of course, if you know for sure that your partner is fooling around, that's another matter and it should be faced and dealt with.

A trick that I have used, with a good deal of success, is to use the international "no" sign to circle and slash any thoughts I want to dismiss. I keep that visualization in place until all the negativity is gone. I also pay more attention to how I speak. I avoid phrases like "to die for," "it's killing me," or "it's driving me crazy." These thoughts, once verbalized, get internalized as fact. Often the body can't detect what is just a saying and what is actually happening.

I feel that in order to really live a healthy, happy, and fulfilled life—in other words, in order to get well—you have to evaluate every aspect of your personal environment. Look at your relationships, your job, and how you spend your free time. Which people and situations are contributing to your peace of mind and which aren't? It is all too easy to stay in a situation because it is familiar, and familiar patterns are hard to break. When I was in the hospital a friend sent me a card that read, "We cannot change unless we survive, and we will not survive unless we change." The two are interdependent and equally challenging. Neither happens overnight.

Lifestyle modification can be accomplished only in small increments. Otherwise we give up. I read once that habit is not to be flung out the window but to be coaxed down the stairs one step at a time. Before we can even begin the coaxing, however, we need to have a clear idea of what is and is not working for us. Unfortunately, too many of us spend too little time trying to find answers to those questions. Even if we do, we often lose sight of the fact that the answers change as we enter different stages in our lives. In the wellness group I often planned exercises that would lead us to think in an enjoyable way about simple pleasures and simple needs. Who was it that said, "Life isn't a matter of milestones, but of moments"?

One of the early assignments that I presented to the group was for each of us to write down, in the form of a poem, the small things that bring us joy, that keep us centered. Those who took the time to sit down and give it some serious thought learned a thing or two about how to enrich their lives. Of course, not only does one have to record these revelations, one has to act on them. One woman in the group noted that what she enjoyed the most in the world was to sit by the fireplace with a cup of hot choco-late. She had all the elements—cocoa, coffee cups, a chair, a fire-place, wood—but couldn't somehow find twenty minutes to pull it off.

My personal insights, which I try to refer to frequently and take to heart, are as follows:

> *When I think of nourishment, of nurturing myself, I think of the quiet beauty of nature . . . wildflowers in bloom, fluffy cumulus clouds playing hide-and-seek with the sun, the majesty of the mountains, and the soothing rhythms of the sea; I think of my home, my husband, and my dog, of cuddling under the covers with a good book; I think of my dear friends: Sally with her unfailing strength, humor, and insights . . . of Mary Brent and her bountiful love, of Nancy and her loyal friendship . . . I think of spontaneous laughter, the sound of wind chimes . . . a quiet, romantic dinner. . . . I think of my sister Lisa—so much like me but always childlike, always play-ful, full of life . . . I think of my father and his successful quest for enlightenment, his knowledge, his strength. . . . I think of unexpected gifts, new and old friends, the twin-kle of fireflies, and the flutter of hummingbirds.*

Some poets write of living differently if given the choice—less work, fewer beans, and of course the popular, "When I am an old woman I shall wear purple. . . ." It seems to me to be a good thing to think about before it's too late.

I suggested to the other women in our support group that we try it. "What would you do if you had no obligations? No one looking over your shoulder saying you should or shouldn't? What would you do? Where would you be? What fantasies would you indulge?"

I personally gave a lot of thought to those questions, and this was the result:

When I Am an Old Woman. . . . by Laura Evans

I shall dye my hair red and wear high-top basketball shoes. I shall wear silk scarves and rhinestone pins with my sweats. I shall wear a different perfume every day and sport mod sunglasses. I'll get a tattoo.

I shall get a post office box under an alias and place ridiculous ads in the personals column just to read the results. I'll write a book of nonsense or fact or both.

I will shoot my scale and make chocolate chip cookies and shamelessly eat all the dough. I will stay up all night watching old movies and sleep with all of my stuffed animals—at once.

I will go for walks at 3:00 A.M., then sleep until noon.

I'll make boxes covered with buttons and glitter and fake gemstones and give them as gifts.

I will learn to rap-dance and speak Swahili.

I will go to a séance and buy a Ouija board.

I will rent an old cabin in the woods, hole up with my dog, and write to everyone I've ever known. Then I will sleep outside and count the stars and think about what color I should dye my hair next.

The purpose of the exercise, of course, is to see if, perhaps, there are things you want out of life—things that would make you happier—that you should go ahead and do now. No time like the present. Be prepared, however, for others not sharing the urgency you feel for your own plans.

Roger was genuinely dismayed when I announced my intention of following through with one of my fantasies.

"I'm going to get a tattoo," I announced one evening.

"You're what?" he quickly responded.

"I'm going to get a tattoo," I reiterated.

"You're not serious." He looked at me sideways.

"Yes, I am."

"Have you thought this out?" he questioned, hoping I hadn't gone off the deep end. "They're permanent. Are you sure you want something that will be there forever? It might seem like a good idea now, but will you like it five or ten years from now?"

The conservative voice of caution. I only smiled. Roger knew me well. I went out on a limb a lot, but he also knew that once I made up my mind, it was a done deal. Nothing would dissuade me.

I decided to get my tattoo when I returned to San Francisco for my next full checkup. I figured I could use a personal treat after a day of blood tests, bone scan, chest X ray, mammogram, and so forth. I mentioned it casually in conversation one evening with my good friend Sally Chapman.

"Oh, by the way, I'm thinking of getting a tattoo," I tossed out.

"You what?" Sally screamed.

"A tattoo, you know—"

"Yes, I know, I know! I just can't believe it. I've always wanted a tattoo," she interrupted.

"You're kidding," I responded, only half surprised. We were so much alike.

"No, of course not!" came her immediate reply.

"There is a place in San Francisco, Lyle Tuttle's tattoo parlor, that is infamous. I was going to try and make an appointment around my next doctor's appointment in February. Do you want to go with me?"

"Of course I do!"

We spent the next four months perusing tattoo magazines and looking in library books at different symbols. We had both decided that we wanted something unique, something that had particular meaning in each of our lives. Once that decision was made, we had to figure out where the tattoo would be placed on our bodies.

In the interim, we also had to humor our spouses, neither of whom totally believed that we were going to go through with this.

Sally met me in San Francisco on a clear, crisp Friday afternoon. Her husband, Jack, had come with her so that he could commiserate with Roger while we "foolishly mutilated our bodies." The plan was to meet for dinner afterward, which never panned out since our project took the better part of the evening.

Lyle's parlor was not hard to find. The exterior looked as if it, like the regulars who came there, had succumbed repeatedly to needle and ink. Numerous colorful drawings flanked the entrance, which was guarded by a cardboard cutout of a very muscular, tattooed sailor. We stood there staring for a moment before taking a deep breath and heading inside.

Neither of us had been in a place like this before, of course, and there was a moment of concern as to whether we really belonged there. We nervously looked around the studio. It was a small room no bigger than most modest motel rooms. The walls were all decorated with multicolored hearts and snakes, American flags, women with bare breasts, and vicious looking dragons. Racks of designs, most of which looked vaguely like ones I had seen on the few Hell's Angels who had passed my way, were displayed in the center of the room. We were thankful we had brought our own designs.

Floating between the walls and the central exhibit were Mr. Tuttle regulars, we assumed, judging from the elaborate ornamentation on most of their bodies. I also noticed pink hair, a nose ring, and a heavily spiked hairdo that stood eight inches straight up in the air. Sally and I, in our slacks and blazers and softly coiffed hair, definitely did not look like we were in the right place.

As if sensing the same thing, one of the tattooers looked up from the body he had been working on. "Can I help you two girls?"

"Yes, we, ah, called about an appointment," we answered together.

"Oh yeah, Evans and Chapman. Hang on for a bit. I'll be about twenty minutes. Have you decided what you want?" he asked out of the side of his mouth, as he went back to work.

"Yes, we have," we said with a confidence that barely masked our unease.

While we waited, we watched.

We peered over the waist-high counter and observed Lyle's right-hand man gingerly put the final touches on a mural of a strange and detailed forest scene on a woman's back. Judging from how long these were supposed to take, he must have been working on this one for weeks. The last tree, flower, and bird were almost in place. The woman was motionless.

"Do you think she's dead?" I asked Sally.

"No, you're not supposed to move," Sally answered quietly.

"Then, since she's so quiet, maybe it doesn't hurt."

Sally laughed nervously. Neither of us was scared or a stranger to pain, but there's always that anticipation.

We were also beginning to think that our choices were a little conservative. Sally, a Florida resident, had picked a delicate orange blossom, and I had sketched a somewhat larger, but still very civilized, bear totem.

We grew tired of watching as Lee completed his handiwork. Instead we looked at dragons and skulls and naked ladies.

"Next," Lee announced as the mural-woman got up to leave.

"You go first," Sally said.

"No, you. Mine will take longer," I quickly responded. Both of us secretly wanted to be first so we wouldn't have to watch the other go through it, not knowing how much pain our friend would have to endure.

"Who is it, then?" asked Lee. No doubt he'd seen this kind of behavior before.

"Okay, I'll go," said Sally.

"First time, huh?" Lee asked as he positioned Sally on the table.

Lee went to work on Sally's shoulder while I stood by the counter. I offered my friend what moral support I could, but my knees got weak every time she grimaced. Although I didn't like pain, I knew I could handle it, but I hated to see anyone suffer, especially someone I cared about. Plus, I would rather have gotten on with something uncomfortable without having to watch a preview of what it was going to be like.

After an hour it was my turn. I lay quietly while Lee etched a bear just above my ankle. It wasn't really painful, just annoying, like a bee poking around with its stinger trying to find the perfect spot to deposit its poison. Mine took almost an hour and a half, and by the time he had finished, I concluded that probably one tattoo was enough. We each paid our one hundred dollars and left bandaged up, with strict instructions not to get that area sweaty or wet for at least three weeks.

The next day Sally went home proudly to Fort Pierce with her new orange blossom. She was sure her sons would be amazed at what Mom had done now, and she devilishly looked forward to the first cocktail party with her reserved friends, where she could wear an off-the-shoulder dress. I returned home to Sun Valley with pretty much the same thing in mind. I loved my beautiful reddish brown bear with his lopsided grin and feather-draped burden and looked forward to showing it off.

The reactions I got should not have been surprising.

"But it's a scar," one of my friends reminded me.

"Perhaps, but it's one I chose, and I happen to think it's pretty," I said in defense.

"But you'll have to look at it for your whole life," someone else responded.

That was the clincher, and it endeared my bear to me even more. "If I have to look at this for another fifty years, I'll be one happy camper," I replied with an ear-to-ear grin, effectively ending that conversation.

Years ago I would have never gotten a tattoo, would never have considered it. The fact that it's a tattoo is not even the issue. The issue is, rather, that I changed my mind. I allowed myself to look at things differently, from another angle, another perspective—in this case, less seriously. In a way I became like the patient who said to his doctor, "I didn't come to be told I'm burning the candle at both ends, I came for more wax." My flame was still burning, but now with more playfulness, no longer in out-of-control busyness.

■ ■ ■

I am a great believer in lists. I recommend that people write everything down in black and white. Otherwise things tend to float around the cerebellum getting bumped into and pushed aside. I'm talking about itemizing not what's in the kitchen but what's in your head. I suggest an inventory of what makes you angry, fearful, sad, excited, joyous, proud. What you don't like about yourself and what makes you the good, unique individual that you are. What you can do well and what you really don't have an aptitude for. Somewhere in the maze will be the spark of a new direction that could provide fulfillment you never thought you would have. I know it has worked for me.

A recurring theme on my feel-good lists is a deep-rooted affection for animals. I have always felt that much can be learned from our furry counterparts. Like most humans, they spend their whole lives in the survival mode, but I feel they handle it much better than we do. After my illness, we brought an animal into our lives, and he taught me about building bridges from my old life to my new in ways I never would have anticipated.

CHAPTER 13

Animal Lessons

There are two ways of spreading light:
To be the candle or the mirror that reflects it.

Anaïs Nin

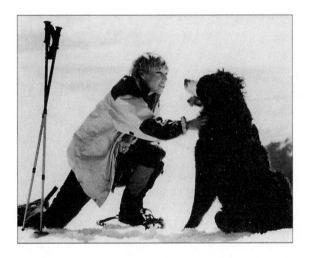

I didn't feel I could have a family and a career and do both well. Besides, I had this foreboding mental picture of the cover of a Life magazine, "Lucky mother gives birth to six healthy babies," with me looking forlorn in the background. I also felt that I was capable of loving too much and that if I ever lost a child I'd be destroyed.

———————■———————

In March of 1995 I learned that our dog, Buster, had cancer, at the age of four and a half. What a cruel joke. I was pained beyond belief. He was my buddy, my companion, my sweet boy.

Roger and I had owned a dog years ago, a beautiful springer spaniel. When we had moved from Denver to Boston, to an inner-city house, we had sent our two-year-old pup to live with Roger's brother in California. Sadly enough, Clancy had run under the tires of a van shortly after he arrived there. It took a while, almost twelve years, before we were ready for another animal. Now Roger, in particular, felt that a pet would be a good companion for me as I built back from the cancer and the treatment.

However, Dr. Lyding, who had supervised my bone marrow transplant, was not too keen on the idea.

"Wait a couple of months," Dr. Lyding insisted in our final conversation after the treatment, a couple of days before we headed back to Idaho. "Your immune system isn't strong enough to get a pet yet."

So we waited two months. Our choice was a Bernese mountain dog. We had first been introduced to the breed in Switzerland and had been charmed by the big furry countenances and happy-go-lucky faces of the Bernese. Sun Valley seemed like a perfect alpine setting for one of our own.

After many phone calls and previewing a snapshot, Buster came into our lives. He arrived with his brother from Colorado in a small shipping crate at the Salt Lake City airport. The two tiny bundles of fur were hungry and thirsty. One of these fur balls would stay with us, and the other would find his new home with a good friend of ours. I carried Buster on my lap the whole drive home, six hours to Sun Valley. His soft little head was pressed to my bosom, the child I never had. I knew instantly that this fuzzy little guy would get me well, that I would rely on him and he on me. Somehow, together, we would find the solutions to all the unanswered questions that rattled around in my mind. My husband had been tremendously supportive, putting aside his work and his own grief to be there for me. But some things I would have to figure out on my own, like where I fit into this new life and how to mesh who I was before with who I was becoming. Now I knew that I would be able to work things out, with the help of this petite package.

The tiny tyke grew quickly into a gentle, full-sized 115-pound animal. The fleece bed we bought him soon became his pillow. He'd lie on it at night at the head of our bed, quietly but intently kneading the pile back and forth, suckling the soft fleece like a mother's tit with his strong front paws.

In the mornings Buster would wake me with his tongue, seeking out the toes that would inevitably be sticking out from underneath the sheet. If I wasn't ready to get up, I would simply reply, "Not yet, Big Boy," and he would plop back down with a sigh.

When Roger was away, I would sometimes sleep on the floor with Buster's body warm against mine, my arm draped over his shoulders, or I would sit watching old movies with Big Boy's head in my lap, content as I caressed his ears. For the first two years, I groomed him every night, later twice a week, lavishing him with attention.

"I want to come back as Buster," Roger commented enviously one night. "He gets more attention than anybody." Which was not hard to understand if you ever saw our sweet boy.

Buster had a face painted by angels. A wide white blaze cut a swath down his forehead and wrapped around his chin. Perky, rust-colored eyebrows framed large brown marble eyes and would move up and down his forehead, Groucho Marx–style, measuring the meaning of my words. Eager to understand, he would tilt his head, often until it was nearly parallel to the floor, as if the words might trickle down into his ears and make more sense. He was a quick learner, as it was, and we were soon spelling t-r-e-a-t and a few other of his favorite words.

In me, our dog had a good, methodical teacher. Wherever I went, he was by my side. And I would always talk to him slowly, enunciating every word carefully, repeating myself so he would remember.

"I swear Buster speaks English," my friend Kristy had commented one afternoon in my office. "He knows everything we're saying."

It is difficult to explain the appeal of Bernese mountain dogs to someone who doesn't know the breed. One story, however, sums it up for me. A woman was inside her house when she was brutally attacked by a burglar. Her Berner, witnessing this from the outside, crashed through the plateglass window, scaring off the intruder and saving his owner's life. The dog then sat mournfully in the corner, feeling bad for having broken the window.

Knowing what I do now about Bernese mountain dogs, I'm sure the story is accurate.

Although Berners have their own unique personalities, they show the same endearing loyalty that most dogs display. As a poster on our bathroom wall reads, "Dogs invented unconditional love." One young woman captured the essence of that affection in the description of the look her dog gives her when she comes home from work: "Oh, God, you're home. You are so great. You are the center of my universe. I love you. *Please* let me kiss you." I imagine that Buster was no more loyal or loving than any other pet, but he did have an especially sweet nature, and of course he was my boy.

Buster was with me practically twenty-four hours a day. He would sit loyally next to my desk in the office or tied up out front at the athletic club, or he would escort me on occasional shopping trips. When I had to leave town, I would call home every night checking up on Roger and our dog. After we finished talking, my husband would press the phone against Buster's ear and I would tell our buddy how much I loved him. In return, my husband later told me, Buster would lick the receiver.

Buster was well known in Sun Valley, not just for his size and his antics, but also for his almost regal demeanor and his huge, perfectly marked head. He has indirectly been the cause of a growing number of Berners in town. But as one young girl noted, "Buster is still the king."

Buster's picture even hangs in our local bank, taken the day he scared silly someone who didn't know him. It really was the tellers' fault, since they could not resist plying Buster with treats when we visited. That particular day Buster made a beeline for the closest teller, plopping his sizable paws on the counter, stretching himself to his full five and a half feet, and in the process knocking over some poor, unsuspecting customer. All the guy saw as he let out a terrified yelp was a black furry monster. The bemused teller tried to lighten the situation by explaining, "It's only Buster, he's come in for his withdrool."

Buster and I hiked together, and he quickly gained the dubious distinction of being my personal trainer. If I was in the office and started to get overwhelmed, I would turn to Buster. "Okay, Buster, that's it. We're out of here. I can either make myself sick dealing with all this stuff, or we can go for a hike." Buster would always jump up in agreement, *hike* being one of his favorite words. Every day he would wait patiently in my office, longing to hear that word. Once on the trail, I would watch him ahead of me, glancing back occasionally to make sure I was coming. I would smile at his unrestrained joy. And I would marvel at the size of him, 115 pounds, the size of a person, and how softly he walked, barely touching the ground. Often I would look down at the loose dirt in search of his prints, finding only shallow indentations where his paws had landed. "If only I could do that," I would say to myself. "That will be my goal, starting today, to walk softly, to rid my mind of all that weighs heavily." I remembered Bernie Siegel's message from God, which Bernie offered as the finale of the talk that I attended: "Never, never, never, ever, ever carry the weight of the world on your shoulders. That is my job." Buster must have already gotten the message.

On one spring foray into the hills behind our house, I misjudged the condition of the terrain. "Buster, I may be in trouble here," I heard myself saying. Ten feet down the icy slope, Buster's eyebrows raised a quarter of an inch, his eyes burning into mine, his always smiling mouth flat against his jaw. I looked down at my sneakers, mud covered and worn from miles of backcountry travel. "How could I have been so stupid? It is only April, too early in the spring to be out in the mountains without hiking boots, at least." Furthermore, I had been daydreaming. Foolishly, I had been mulling over what I would do with the twenty-million-dollar lottery jackpot if my numbers came in, oblivious to the ground underfoot, which had changed from mud to snow to ice.

To ease my discomfort, I continued my one-sided conversation. "You may have to help me, big guy," I spoke, out loud. "I could slip all the way to Hailey." I stared ahead at the slick trail, trying to decide whether to turn back or to continue forward.

Before I even saw him move, Buster was by my side, positioned above me on the slope, his mouth gently cradling my uphill arm, his eyes searching mine. I loved this boy. He was my only child, my animal soul mate.

In the winter we would go snowshoeing, Buster in the lead, escaping the decadent madness of the holiday season and letting the serene beauty of the mountains and wilderness soothe our spirits. We would tromp through the blanket of white diamond-like snow, glistening as if strewn with millions of gems, around corners into a treasure chest of valleys and trees sugar-coated with the new-fallen flakes. It is there that I would feel most alive, most at peace, reveling in the ever-changing, ever-beautiful majesty of nature.

It was no different for Buster. I could see it in the bounce in his step, the twinkle in his eyes, the smile that played on his lips as he turned his head in my direction as if to say, "Thank you, Mom, this works for me, but hurry up because there's so much to see and smell." Then he would roll over, upside down in the snow, checking to make sure I was watching and that the distance between us hadn't gotten too small. God forbid that I should overtake my Big Boy!

His bravado, of course, was all a big hoax. Buster was about as brave as a rabbit. I'd seen him jump six-foot snowbanks to get out of the reach of dogs one-tenth his size. He'd scurry out of the room and up the stairs if someone picked up a match to light a fire. I'd even spied him lifting his leg to pee—the front one, though, letting fly all over his back leg. But his goofy, unaggressive nature is one of the things that endeared Big Boy most to me—that and his gentle spirit. When I was sad, he was always there.

One night the two of us were seated on the floor of the bedroom watching old home movies—yet another reminder of how things change—when I found myself crying, wishing I could resurrect my carefree days before cancer. Buster moved closer to me, cocking his head, hoping to soothe me with his presence. "It's okay, sweet boy," I said between sobs, looking into his concerned eyes. "I love you, angel boy. I'm just sad and confused. I want my old life back." Buster lifted up his head, reached up with his tongue, and licked the tears off my face, in the process cleansing my dispirited soul. Buster made me forget the sadness, the upheaval, the overwhelming loss I sometimes felt for the life I had left behind.

One night while grooming our sweet boy, I found four or five lumps on his head. I wasn't overly concerned. *It's probably doggy measles,* I remember thinking. But I had it checked out anyway. To be on the safe side, our vet took an X ray of Buster's lungs. It never occurred to me that our dog might really be sick, so when Dr. Acker called with the test results, I was shocked. "Laura, Buster has three large tumors on his lungs. He has a rare form of cancer called malignant histiosytosis that attacks the lymph system first, then the organs. I am sorry." I know I stopped breathing. How could this possibly be? He wasn't even five years old. And why such a dear sweet soul like our Big Boy? Why cancer? It would almost have been easier on me if he had been hit by a car. I had dealt enough with cancer.

Within a month, the cancer had spread to Buster's brain and he went blind in one eye. I couldn't contain my sadness. It came in sudden waves—a quick blow to the stomach, my breath catching in my throat, tears filling my eyes.

In an effort to save his life, we put Buster on chemotherapy. He stoically accepted the catheter while I cringed, remembering, feeling again the death-red drugs course through my own veins. He took three treatments of the drugs, but it was useless. Buster was weakening, and it broke my heart.

There was one hope. A month before Buster was diagnosed, I had been in Philadelphia meeting with the Wistar Institute, the oldest cancer research facility in the country. While I was there, they had talked enthusiastically about their "killer cell" program. These cells, present in all of us, are able to seek out and destroy disease. The scientists had been increasing the number of killer cells in cancer-infected rats and were finding it to be an effective means of wiping out tumors without damaging any good cells. They had also recently had success in curing a dog that was terminally ill with the disease. Ironically, I had jokingly commented, "Well, if my dog ever gets cancer, I'm bringing him here."

After several subsequent conversations, my husband and I started making plans to drive Buster to Philadelphia. The researchers at Wistar were pleased to have our Big Boy available to further their research. Even after the chemo and a fifteen-pound weight loss, our dog was still a hundred times bigger than the rats they had been working on. If the killer cells could save his life, we would be that much closer to a cure in humans. And we would have our dog back.

I was still afraid, afraid of losing my buddy. I would have to avert my eyes when the sadness rolled over me, because Buster could see it and would know that something was terribly wrong. I muscled up, knowing he was still with me, not wanting to mourn his death until he was gone. When I did look into his eyes, however, I thought I saw pain. Yet I know it was merely a reflection of my own. For the first time I understood how Roger felt, and Mom, my sisters, and close friends, looking at me through the plastic of my bubble, feeling the agony I now felt, watching hopelessly, wishing to turn back the clock to change things somehow. All of us were trying to brace ourselves to be able to deal with the emptiness, the sadness, the unfairness of it all. Often we lose sight of the fact that the one battling the illness doesn't suffer the same emotional trauma as those on the outside looking in.

It had been six weeks since Buster's diagnosis when Wistar called with unsettling news. "We won't have enough cells ready for a month," Dr. Jeglum informed me. "A month?" *A month! Not that long. Buster's one chance for survival out the window.* Buster didn't have a month. I realized how much I had been counting on this procedure. A clinical test, like I had gone through, that would save him and in the process make him part of a larger cure.

As I hung up the phone, I remembered Christmas and Buster's stocking, which had hung from the mantel for the last three years. I had spent weeks making it, cutting out little felt bones and a red fire hydrant and a likeness of Big Boy with his ever-present scarf around his neck. Would it ever hang on the fireplace again?

I remembered one of my friends telling me, "Understand that dogs don't know they're dying. Only people know that and fear death." It didn't alleviate my sadness one bit.

It was almost spring, but the new season was tainted for me with the reality of the loss I would no doubt have to face. Nevertheless, I needed to get into the wilderness to remind myself of all the beauty that still existed. I stepped around the patches of snow as I headed up the ski mountain, enjoying the sun, tired of the dreary rain of the last week. The first robins were out, fat and sassy, digging around on the hillsides. Although it felt good to be outside, I was lonely and sad. I couldn't stop thinking about Buster, and I realized that this was my first hike without him. Except for steep or particularly long climbs, he had always been by my side, more or less, thrilled to be out-of-doors, away from it all, mirroring my sentiments exactly. Buster had helped me see nature through his eyes. Every twig, every rock, leaf, and flower, was a marvel in itself. Every moment in the wilderness was an adventure. In his own way Buster would laugh out loud, bounding through bushes and patches of wildflowers, circling back if I was slow. He would happily dunk his body in high mountain lakes, immune to the cold water, cooling off after the long hike. But those days were over.

Within another week Buster went completely blind. I first realized this driving home from work. It was so quiet in the back of the car that I checked the rearview mirror. Buster was seated, tilting his head in all directions, his eyes searching the back of the Jeep, looking for something, anything, finding only darkness. I gripped the steering wheel and let out a moan. My poor, sweet boy.

Despite his blindness, Buster was still robust and had the same spark he'd always had. But now he would bounce around, bumping into things, until he would hit a spot where his sense of smell or will couldn't move him forward. Then he was lost, unsure of where he was or where to go, standing quietly, scared, confused, and disoriented by the blackness that surrounded him.

I knew what he was experiencing. I have felt that way, at times, rebuilding from my illness, frozen, totally immobile, at a loss as to which way to turn, overwhelmed by everything in my life. But I snap out of it, as Buster did, focusing on one small thing to point me in the right direction. Big Boy, out of necessity, learned a new way to walk, lifting up his front paw, feeling for obstacles, then setting it on the ground, his indomitable spirit pushing him forward.

I thought of our dog in healthier days and remembered our vet saying, "Buster makes you laugh. What more could you ask from a pet?"

And he did, daily. On my kitchen wall is a sign that reads, "The most wasted day of all is that on which you have not laughed." With Buster I never had to look for the laughter.

"Dogs are angel guides to help us through the tough times," a friend told me in those final days. Buster had been my guide. I hadn't known when I was sick that he was out there for me to help me rebuild my life. His spirit was a rare and wonderful gift. I could not imagine life without his special energy, and there were times I had wondered if I could go on if anything happened to him. He was that closely tied to my wellness. But I had to deal with the fact that Buster was indeed dying, bit by bit, being eaten up from the inside by the same insidious disease that had tried to claim my life.

Buster was totally blind for only two days. The last Friday of April, with the assistance of our vet, Randy Acker, we put him to sleep by the river, in the wilderness he so loved. He died peacefully in our arms, one last treat in his mouth, the quiet surroundings interrupted only by my wails, a realization of the sudden emptiness of a space that only he could fill.

Buster did not suffer, did not deteriorate to the point that life no longer held beauty for him. He died with dignity as he lived his life. How very much I hope to go the same way, when I know the sun is fading but I can still feel the last rays of its warmth.

Buster's energy was powerful. He was such a positive force. When he took his last breath, it had been five years since I was diagnosed with breast cancer. He had helped to heal me. Now I choose to believe that his vitality had moved on to help someone else. I don't dismiss the comment that several people made, "Buster took your cancer."

Later that spring, the weather turned warm, and Roger and I started hiking in the hills surrounding Sun Valley. We would go to all of Buster's favorite places, taking his energy with us and spreading his ashes on the summits. Often I hiked alone, talking to Buster as if he were there again beside me. Always I carried the small plastic tube that contained a portion of his remains. One day in particular stands out in my mind. It was just Buster and I and the incomparable beauty of a clear, sunny day in the mountains.

"You would have liked this, Big Boy," I mentioned aloud. "What a glorious day." I continued up, hiking through knee-deep wildflowers in vibrant shades of purple, yellow, orange, and blue. I would stop occasionally, looking for the perfect spot to leave my sweet boy. "No, not yet. Higher, where the views are 360 degrees. You always did like to be on top, sort of like your mom."

We continued our ascent until I spotted a small bush on the top of a steep ridge that was framed on all sides by mountains and valleys. "Perfect. This will do," I decided as I pulled the plastic tube from around my neck. Opening it, I announced to the wind, "I love you, Big Boy," and flung his ashes over my head. As I did, my heart caught in my throat and tears brimmed in the corners of my eyes. "I miss you, Buster." Just then, I heard my name.

"Laura." I looked around. There was nobody up here. Where could that voice be coming from?

"Laura," I heard a second time. It sounded like Roger, but it couldn't be. "Hello," I shot back. I'm sure I heard someone calling my name. I looked up into the wooded area behind me. Was someone up there? Suddenly, a solitary antelope came bounding out of the trees toward me, leaping through the air like a sleek rabbit. The antelope passed within ten feet of where I stood and then disappeared into the woods below. I was awestruck, unable to move, taken aback by what had just happened. "Was that you, Big Boy?" I wondered aloud. Whatever had occurred was a gift— a precious, unforgettable, spiritual gift of fabulous animal energy. So alive.

A Soviet Summit

Climbing is not a battle with the elements, nor against the law of gravity; it's a battle against oneself.

Walter Bonatti

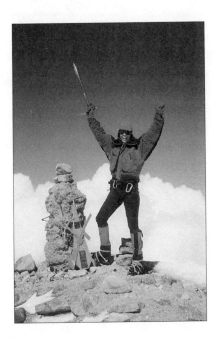

Climbing is a reconfirmation of one's own strength and ca-
pacity to survive. To climb mountains, in itself, enriches our
lives. It opens doors, expands our awareness, and exposes
us to new and enlightening experiences.

———————■———————

We had heard all the horror stories surrounding Aeroflot
Airlines. More accidents than any other carrier in the
world, never on time, poorly maintained, independently owned
and operated, with no central checks and balances for safety.
None of this information was very reassuring. Twelve of us, from
almost as many different states, were to take several Aeroflot
flights before reaching our final destination, Mount Elbrus in the
Caucasus mountain range in southeast Russia. Although Elbrus
is the highest mountain in Europe, the transportation getting
there was more unnerving than the prospect of the climb itself.

But I had been intrigued with Russia for a long time, so the
risks didn't matter. Sort of like the forbidden fruit. I had been
weaned on James Bond movies and the notion that Russians were
the big, bad enemy. And over the years I had met many Russian
immigrants who became close friends and spoke of the beauty of
their homeland and how I must one day go there. What better
way than to climb, especially if it meant the possibility of reaching another of the seven continental summits?

In the hospital, looking out at the park, I would daydream
about climbing the continental summits. At least six of them,

anyway. I would picture myself on the top, hale and hearty, without a care in the world, following my desire. Of course, it didn't seem at all realistic, but that didn't matter. The concept kept me going.

I had recently read Frank Wells and Dick Bass's account of their quest to climb the highest mountain on each of the seven continents. They were successful, and their book, *Seven Summits*, whetted the appetite of many experienced and novice climbers to try the same thing. For me, to be able to climb *any* of the continental summits was a dream come true.

In addition to loving climbing, I loved to travel. My parents were both professors, with their summers free, allowing the family long periods of time for excursions. We often went to Michigan to see my grandparents, but we also spent an eye-opening summer in northern California during the zenith of the Haight-Ashbury counterculture. Another memorable summer was spent traveling around Mexico living with local families and visiting the grand cities of Guadalajara and Mexico City. Having grown up in a small town in Ohio, I was vastly curious about distant places, which I was certain would be infinitely more interesting than where I was from.

Russia certainly qualified. And I wasn't disappointed.

We had a day of leisure in Moscow before our feared Aeroflot flights. It was mostly spent wandering around Gorky Park and Red Square, the vast courtyard in front of the Kremlin. I couldn't begin to count the number of times I had seen these impressive arenas in *Newsweek* and on television, so it was a surreal experience to all of a sudden be there, in the picture.

My first impression of Russia and its inhabitants could be summed up in one word: *dour*. A heaviness seemed to permeate everything—the architecture, the clothing, people's voices, the weather. Even the elegant and exotic splendor of Saint Basil's Cathedral, with its many rounded and gilt spires, was tainted with the knowledge that the architect had been blinded after his masterpiece was complete so that it could never be reproduced.

Following a day and a half of sight-seeing, we braved Aeroflot. We were boarded through the rear of the aircraft. And that's exactly what it smelled like. When I had the unfortunate opportunity of using the bathroom facilities at one point during the flight, I understood why. The toilet was no more than a mile-high outhouse with a hole, no sink, and no toilet paper.

People chose their own seats. I was one of the luckier ones, finding a seat with a backrest that didn't continually flop forward and a seat belt that worked. Once everyone was seated, the steward came through the cabin with a Polaroid, just in case someone wanted to record this momentous occasion. That was followed by a tray of used-looking purses, brushes, and jawbreakers, all evidently for sale.

"I guess that's our in-flight duty-free shopping," I whispered to guide Mark Tucker, who happened to be sitting next to me.

Tuck looked over at me. "Yeah. I was kind of waiting for the part about the safety features of the plane. I guess he slept through that."

On that note, I crossed myself and said a silent prayer as the plane lifted off the ground.

After one more Aeroflot flight we thankfully landed on a dark and mostly deserted runway in a remote corner of Russia. We were pleased to see a bus waiting to take us to our next accommodations. It took close to an hour, however, to round up all the gear, counting each large duffel to make sure that no one's personal gear or any group gear got left behind.

Once on board the bus, we spread out. It was close to 9:00 P.M. on a dark, moonless night, so we rolled up our jackets, wedged them between the windows and our heads, and prepared for a little shut-eye. We finally felt like we could relax. However, we had not traveled far before the bus driver pulled over to the side of the road. Our only local, bilingual climber got off, and we heard whispered voices in Russian. Tuck and Robert Link, our two Summits guides, were instantly on alert, as were we all. We listened, for what seemed an eternity but was probably no more than ten minutes, to the unintelligible words.

Looking out the window at the bleak and foreign landscape, we strained to see what was going on. We had heard stories of the Russian Mafia and only hoped that they weren't taking an interest in us. It hadn't really occurred to us that prior to the climb Aeroflot would not be our only risk.

As suddenly as he had disembarked, our Russian climber re-boarded and we were again moving. Nothing was said. I looked at the wary faces around me and knew that sleep was now out of the question. We had no idea what had just transpired, but there had been an undercurrent of danger. Once more we were stopped, and we all sat at attention, bracing ourselves for whatever might come. As before, after a lengthy, hushed conversation, we silently moved on. We were later informed that those were unauthorized but highly respected toll stops, taken seriously by anyone who was requested to pull over. Tariffs had to be negotiated, questions answered. How many people, what nationality, what are they doing here?

There was a collective sigh of relief when we reached the gate to the Dacha, an inn that would be our home for the few days before and after the climb. As we wound our way up the long tree-lined driveway to the entrance, we were pleased to note that our new residence had a secure and secluded atmosphere. This feeling was reinforced when Robert informed us that the estate had once been frequented by the kingpins of the Communist Party. No doubt for them safety had been a major consideration.

After wearily unloading our heavy duffels, we were delighted to find that our rooms were oversized suites. Each contained two beds, a desk, an armoire, end tables with lamps, and a full bath with sink, shower/tub, and toilet. The furniture was vintage 1930s, and we later realized that the plumbing didn't always work, but we made ourselves right at home anyway. We were just happy to be out of Moscow, off Aeroflot, off the bus, and safely ensconced in our own private hideaway.

The following morning, after a hot breakfast served by the staff of the inn, I walked around the grounds, enjoying the solitude. I am always introspective before a climb, not so much because of the inherent dangers in mountaineering, but because I don't know for sure how I'll do. Will I have a problem with altitude? Although I never have before, altitude sickness can strike anyone anytime. Even though I have trained like mad, hiking as much as five and six hours a day, will I be strong? And there was always the nagging memory of my very first Rainier climb and the resulting injury.

I'll be fine, I decided, summoning up my strength, putting aside any doubts or misgivings. I took a few deep breaths, preparing my lungs for what lay ahead.

I strolled leisurely, allowing myself to take in the surroundings. The property was nestled in a narrow valley circled by rock-strewn hills and covered with a dense thicket of evergreen trees. A five-foot-wide river roared down from those hills through the edge of the property. Boulders lined the banks of the river, providing a nice platform on which to lounge and watch the water as it spiraled past the Dacha, washing over rocks and felled branches on its way. I continued walking for perhaps a half a mile, when I reached a fence that was clearly the boundary for the domain.

In my reverie, I failed to notice an armed guard, in full military attire, on the opposite side of the fence. By the time I felt his presence, we were no more than five feet apart and I found myself staring into two of the most inhospitable eyes I have ever seen. My gaze drifted to the rifle he was holding, which suddenly seemed to be clutched tighter than a second before. Almost as a reflex, I turned, not suddenly but deliberately. As I walked away, I prayed. What I had just seen was hatred. Pure, unmasked hatred. I felt my back muscles tighten. I half expected the bullet that I believed would be forthcoming, especially if I made any unexpected moves or if the soldier just could not resist. *Guess the cold war isn't completely over after all,* I mulled as I walked. Once back in the protective walls of the Dacha, I resolved not to take any more excursions.

In fact, I was ready to get on with the climbing of Elbrus. Russia was beginning to make me a little nervous. I was pleased when the following day was spent hiking around the local ski area. Being in the mountains got us in the climbing mode and gave our bodies a chance to acclimate. The day ended with a hearty meal of ground beef, mashed potatoes, and soup and a good night's sleep. This would be the final hot meal and soft bed before heading to our destination.

Every mountain is different, with its own special charm and beauty. At first glance, Elbrus was no exception. Its twin summits rise above a snow- and lava-covered base that flows sharply down to a lush narrow valley, the recipient of all the glacial runoff. Encircling Elbrus are layers of prominent, jagged peaks, too many to count. There were literally dozens of rock and ice pyramids jutting into and above the clouds.

Unlike with any other climb I knew of, we were to take a gondola up the lower part of the mountain. "It's unclimbable," someone had mentioned. I was thinking that climbing still might be preferable to more of the local transportation. Nonetheless, we crammed our gear and ourselves into one of the tram cars and buried our noses in one another's shoulders as the gondola lifted higher and higher off the ground. Hazarding a look, I estimated we were several thousand feet above the ground. "A long way to drop," someone pointed out.

Once we were off the tram, our group gear, in this case consisting of ropes, food, fuel, crampons, and ice axes, was ferried up to a higher elevation strapped into chair lifts. We had had enough and decided to walk. Too much sitting around and you start to fear that your body won't move when you want it to. Besides, the chairs were rusty and creaked. Nobody felt like pushing their luck any further.

There was much excitement as we made our way up toward base camp, each of us straining to see where we would be staying, what the route must be, the exact location of the summit. This is what we came for after all. Soon we could see the sun reflecting off the sides of the infamous Pruit hut. Built in 1939, the oblong Pruit hut, consisting of three stories of shiny metal, was the fist structure of its kind and very different from the typical (and more natural) mountain lodges made of stone and wood.

"Can you believe that?" asked Ray, a tall, good-looking Floridian.

"Nope," responded Mary Anne, the shortest but possibly the toughest in our group.

"It looks like a futuristic train car that somehow ran off course and landed on the side of the mountain," I added, squinting up at our soon-to-be shelter.

"Certainly isn't your rustic mountain lodge," Ray commented.

Unbelievable, I thought. *A huge silver bullet lodged in the side of this beautiful landscape.*

"What is all the stuff on the ground, around the building?" Mary Anne asked as we got closer.

"Trash," replied Robert Link, our lead guide.

"Trash!" we replied in astonishment.

"Trash," Robert replied again, disdainfully.

Trash it was, and more than I had ever seen in one place, at one time, outside of a garbage dump. Everywhere I looked there were rotted-out stoves, contorted rust-covered chairs, bottles, paper, feces. Endless debris.

"This is sad," I said to myself, wondering where you would even begin to clean this up. It looked as if no one had ever tried to contain their trash. I was at least proud in the knowledge that we would, but it seemed somewhat futile.

Our accommodations were on the third level of the silver bullet. Each of our rooms was a pie-shaped wedge. Together they formed a semicircle on one end of the floor. All but two rooms had bunk beds and were so small you could open the door only wide enough to squeeze in or out. The bathroom facilities were three floors down and outside, a makeshift outhouse with three holes cut into a wooden floor. They deposited one's waste directly onto the glacier fifteen feet below. We found a better solution: door 100, three down from our bedrooms, opened up to nothing but thin air. It was here that we did our business, leaning our butts out as far as possible, holding onto the sides of the building. Someone had previously dug a sizable ditch directly below our improvised facility, which we hoped and assumed would one day be covered over with rock and ice.

One of the biggest hardships in climbing is sleep. Lying awake that night listening to the clank of tin cans being scattered across the glacier, I tried to will myself under. But it was tough. Unless a huge storm came in, tomorrow was the day. I knew we would be up long before the sun and that I would need every ounce of energy I could muster. I would need all my faculties working, on alert lest the weather change or someone slip. Knowing how much I needed the sleep made it harder to get.

"Time to get up," I heard Tuck tell the room next to ours shortly thereafter. At some point I must have actually gotten some rest.

Once the wake-up call is sounded, there is not a moment to waste. Time is of the essence, for everyone's safety. In climbing, it's okay to start up in the dark when you're fresh and eager. It's quite another thing to come down in darkness, tired, thirsty, and hungry, with the momentum of gravity trying hard to pull you off the mountain. There is a safe window of time on every climb, and it needs to be respected.

Most of us had slept in our long underwear, so it was on with a fleece layer, wind pants and jacket, then boots, gaiters, gloves, and hat. A big slug of water, one last pee, something to eat, headlamp adjusted, and out the door.

With the aid of our headlights, we attached ourselves, at thirty-foot intervals, to the already knotted rope, making certain that the locks on our carabiners were secure. One after another, we headed out, waiting until the line in front of us had uncoiled. We maintained a safe distance from the others on the team, in the event someone fell. More than one climber has opted for less rope (less weight) and has ended up buried in a crevasse. The response time if someone falls is merely seconds. With a little more rope, generally, one has enough time to hurl oneself face down into the mountainside, planting crampon points and ice ax deep into the ice. One person, properly anchored, can hold an average rope team of five or six people.

We moved slowly at first, warming up our muscles, fingers, and toes, trying to find a comfortable rhythm. I was conscious of Renata Whitaker in front of me. Renata, no relation to the climbing Whittakers, was a friend of Mary Anne's and a big supporter of the breast cancer cause. But she had little climbing experience, and I watched uneasily as she proceeded up the mountain, irregularly moving both feet, not trying to rest-step at all. It would be a long day for Renata, that's if she even made it.

Every hour we stopped for water and a bite of whatever snacks we had packed along. "How you doing, Renata?" I asked a couple of times. "I'm okay," she would respond. "Just a little tired. I'll be fine."

Conditions were good. The sun came up in a cloudless sky, and the light layer of snow supported by an underlayer of hard pack made for good footing. The route looked direct, maybe even easy, but the pitch was steady. Four hours into the climb, on a fairly steep slope, Renata started to falter. The slack in the rope in front of me would alternately increase, then decrease, then increase as Renata would slow down, then try to catch up, then slow down again. I knew there was no catching up in mountaineering. Once you're wasted, the climb is over.

Link, at the head of the rope, could feel the rope behind him pulling taut.

"Keep the slack steady. Pick up the pace if you need to," he shot back.

"I need to take a break," Renata responded, trying to talk and take in air at the same time.

"We've only been going about twenty minutes," Link replied, still moving.

"I can't. I have to stop," Renata gasped as she sat down.

Two more climbers turned an hour later, and each of them was escorted down by one of our four guides.

We stopped for sandwiches and fruit in the cleavage between the two mounds that make up Elbrus.

"Which way do we go?" I wanted to know, looking up at two sheer walls.

"We work our way up to the left," Link pointed. "It's the steepest part of the climb."

No kidding.

After lunch we headed up the face leading to the top. I focused on my breathing and any sound that might indicate someone had lost his or her footing. I tried to follow in the steps of Mary Anne, who was now in front of me, but our strides were different and the terrain too steep. With each stride, I would lift up my back leg, digging in with my crampons, making sure they had found purchase, before moving on. I looked up to see the crest of the slope only twenty feet away. Almost there, I thought. I *hope* nobody falls on this section. Only seconds later, Mary Anne did.

"Falling!" I yelled as I dropped into the snow. *Mary Anne forgot that part,* I reflected as I kicked in my toe points. I clung there with the cold metal of my ice ax pressing into my shoulder, my cheek forced against the snow. I waited, hoping I wouldn't feel the tug of the rope behind me.

Link had reached the lip of the incline just as I had let out my scream. Without hesitation, he turned, scrambling back to where Mary Anne lay. He then picked her up and practically threw her onto the top. Tuck moved up his rope team, making sure everyone was okay before we continued up.

What we envisioned being the culmination of our climb proved to be a false summit. It was another four hours before we reached the cross that marked the highest point. As we traversed a slight incline that led to the final grade, I thought about previous climbs. Once I reached the summit, I always felt an almost unbearable joy. It seemed incredible that I could do this. That I really was well again and strong. For me, it was such a great sense of accomplishment, knowing how sick and feeble I had been before. I had almost believed, at one time, that I might never be active again.

When we arrived at the top of Elbrus, it was no different. As I stood there with all of Europe stretched below me, I felt genuinely alive, more alive than I had before I was sick, more than ever before. At that moment, I resolved to continue to hone my climbing skills, my body, and my capacity to withstand whatever adversity came my way.

The round-trip climb from the Pruit hut to the summit and back down again took fourteen hours and covered seventeen miles. We dragged into camp shortly after dark, ready to celebrate our survival and hard-earned victory.

On a given climb, you are often thrown in with strangers, others with whom you share a passion for climbing or adventure or travel but little else. You develop a rapport on the mountain because you have to, but usually the group dynamics are such that people generally do not let down their guard. Typically, people are unable to totally release their jealousies, insecurities, and control. The team that climbed Elbrus was different.

Perhaps because of the dangerous nature of the entire trip or the fact that, of the twelve of us, six were men and six women, all close in age—or maybe it was the Russian vodka—we bonded and fired up for a celebration that will long be remembered.

On the bus, returning to the Dacha, we discussed putting together a climbing calendar featuring all male guides.

"In harnesses and boots and nothing else," one of the women said.

"Yeah, Link could be Mr. January, Tuck Mr. March," I pointed out.

"Or we'll find out their birthdays and they can be featured in that month," another female added.

"A different flavor every month," someone giggled.

And on it went, planting a seed for the evening's entertainment. After champagne and several glasses of vodka, I was joined by the five other women climbers in the largest of the suites. There we shed our sweats, stripping down to the bathing suits we had packed in the unlikely event we could locate a hot tub.

"I can't believe we're doing this," Saskia said, pulling up her short bottoms.

"I can, I think this is great," Mary Anne reassured Saskia.

"This is hysterical," I added.

"You look too sexy," Renata told Nancy and me.

"The harness doesn't fit very snugly over a tank suit," Lisa pointed out, tugging at the webbing that circled her waist.

"They are going to die," we agreed in unison.

Fifteen minutes later, scantily clad and roped together, we pranced through the Dacha singing, "If you want my body and you think I'm sexy, come on baby tell me so. . . . If you really love me and you want to take me, come on baby let it show. . . ."

Tuck, the first to see us, turned the color of a ripe tomato and almost gagged, he was laughing so hard. Link and the other male climbers came out to see what all the commotion was about and quickly scattered, making a beeline for their cameras.

They followed us up and down the stairs, snapping away and cracking up over our getups.

In the living room were our translator, three Russian climbers (who had been our extra guides on the mountain), the cook, and various other employees who serviced the residence. Not sure how they would respond, we made a quick pass through. We could hear their amused laughter as we headed to our rooms to get dressed.

Later, one of our Russian counterparts complimented us by saying it was the best show he had ever seen.

Another added, much to our astonishment, that although he had been raised in the Russian army and trained to kill Americans, he could never imagine killing someone like us!

Much later, we got a preview of what our calendar could be like. Winding down after a huge meal and more vodka, we noticed two lights shining through the living room window. Attached to those lights were Tuck and Link in their undershorts and harnesses and huge grins. They had just tied ropes to the roof of the building, attached themselves to the ropes via carabiners and harnesses, then belayed over the side, pushing off with their feet.

That night we shared some of our dreams and hopes. Americans and Russians, only understanding bits and pieces of each other's languages, we understood the common bond of humanity. The humor in the absurd, the satisfaction in accomplishment, the camaraderie in working together, the joy in the rare special moments that make up our lives.

Sitting there basking in the warmth of my fellow human beings, I had no idea that this goodwill would be magnified tenfold on a mountain to come.

———■———

CHAPTER 15

Expedition Inspiration

Whatever you can do, or dream you can, begin it.
Boldness has genius, power, and magic in it.

W. H. Murray

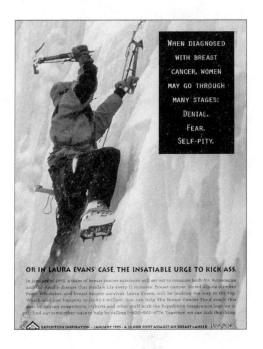

Spiritually, I'm coming home. I am appreciating and savoring all that I am, all that I have, not wanting more, taking nothing for granted. I am going to allow the goodness (God) in me to shine through. I will be more loving. I will use the strength I've gained from my experience with cancer to help others, to help those who need it to realize how much there is to live for.

———■———

In 1983, the first time I met Peter Whittaker, he was doing flips off the back of a boat during a cocktail cruise given by the outdoor gear company JanSport. I was tempted to join him—not that I do much of a flip—but I was on my good behavior, for the following day I would head up Mount Rainier for the first time. Since I had no idea what to expect and wasn't even sure I would make it up the mountain, I felt it would be circumspect to remain low-key. After the climb, of course, it would be another matter.

Of course, I didn't make it to the top that trip, but I have since climbed Rainier many times with Peter as guide. I would never have guessed from that first meeting that Peter and I at a much later date would become involved in a business venture that would change not only our lives but also the lives of many others. After I rebuilt from cancer and started climbing in earnest, I booked several trips with Peter. On these climbs I gained even greater respect for Peter as a mountain guide, and we became good friends. I admired his business acumen and the grounded sensibilities of his beautiful wife, Erika. In the relatively short time that I had known them, they had developed Summits Adventure Travel, one of the more successful adventure travel companies around. Through their rapidly expanding network of guides, Peter and Erika had structured climbs to Africa, Argentina, Antarctica, Bolivia, Ecuador, New Zealand, and Russia. Everyone who went on the Summits trips had a great time, almost always summited, and returned in one piece. Every trip was followed up with a newsletter that made all weekend warriors feel that they were on the inside climbing track.

As Peter and I grew closer, it seemed natural to me that I should make one special request of him—to take my ashes to the top of Rainier. After all, he was young enough to outlive me— that is, if he didn't crack open his head doing back flips off a boat.

We were in the mountains, although I can't seem to remember where, when I asked him. "Peter, this may seem like a strange request and you don't have to do it if you're not comfortable with it, but, ah, when I die, I want my ashes taken to the summit of Rainier. It's recorded in my will. I wondered if you would do this for me."

"I'd be honored," Peter responded without hesitation.

"Well, that's assuming that you don't kick the bucket first," I added, happy to have his commitment but not wanting to dwell too long on the morbidity of the request.

When Roger heard where I wanted my remains, he jokingly responded, "Do you mind if it's a case of Rainier?" But I was serious. The beer wouldn't do. I had taken Dad's ashes up Mount Rainier, and I planned on joining him up there one day.

And there was my great-aunt Ernestine, who had climbed Mount Rainier at the turn of the century. Mom talked about visiting her aunt in Portland when she was ten years old. Ernestine was a strong, flamboyant woman, much different from any women Mom had been around. At night Mom would stay up way past her bedtime, mesmerized by Ernestine's escapades. The one that left the biggest impression was Mount Rainier. In that day and age the idea that women would even consider climbing was foreign. It was equally impossible to imagine the resistance she must have encountered and how awkward it must have been to ascend that huge pile of snow and ice in a skirt. Unfortunately, the only records we have of Ernestine's climb are a few meager diary entries and Mom's recollections. But I know, in my bones, that she was there.

Rainier was the first mountain I ever successfully climbed. Although my initial experience on the mountain was far different from what I had planned, it taught me the difference between discomfort and pain, it taught me how to receive from others and depend on them more, and it most certainly made me tougher. That disappointing outcome also drew me back to the high country. When I returned I fell in love with that magnificent Northwest landmark and became enamored with the sport. Rainier had become part of my destiny, alive or dead, and that's where I wanted my ashes.

During the years following my bout with cancer, I climbed more frequently with Peter and with his company's excellent staff of guides. In addition to Mount Rainier, Kilimanjaro, and Elbrus, I climbed mountains in Mexico and Bolivia. The Mexican volcanoes, Popocatepetl (17,887 feet) and Pico de Orizaba (18,701 feet), provided a natural progression in my plan to climb more and bigger mountains. Each of these climbs could be accomplished in one (approximate) ten-hour day, starting and finishing at an on-mountain lodge. These mountains are also heavily glaciated and offer the opportunity for more practice in mountaineering techniques including rope travel, cramponing, and ice ax rescue.

It was on Orizaba that I first saw Peter spring into action. We were coming down from the summit, trying to keep up a good pace since the winds were howling and snow looked imminent. Bill, in front of me on the rope, was struggling the whole way due to a recent knee injury that probably hadn't had enough time to heal properly.

We knew there were crevasses on Orizaba and had followed a careful route to the top. But, unlike on Rainier, here they were hidden under layers of snow. I was carefully moving downhill, protecting my reconstructed ankle with the weight of my other leg, when I looked up and noticed that Bill had somehow shrunk. I was trying to digest this unusual occurrence when I saw Peter dash from his position at the head of the rope and race back to him.

"What are you guys doing?" he screamed at us. "You should be in an ice ax arrest!" he continued, at the same time extricating Bill from the soft snow that warned of a nearby concealed crevasse. In one fluid blink-of-the-eye movement, Peter had lifted and moved a guy close to fifty pounds heavier than he was. I was impressed not only by Peter's lightning-quick reflexes, but also by the obvious weight of responsibility that rested squarely on his shoulders. It was a mantle that he wore well.

The Mexican volcanoes were followed by a trip to Bolivia and the extraordinarily beautiful Huayna Potosi. At just under 20,000 feet, this impressive peak towers over the surrounding landscape and nestles up against a glistening reservoir.

Two nights would be spent at Zonga Pass, the 15,500-foot base camp, then three on the mountain itself. Unlike my previous climbs, the final 600-foot approach consisted of a fifty- to fifty-five-degree headwall that culminated in a knife-edged summit. It was my first experience with jumars and fixed lines. A continuous line of rope was stretched the six hundred vertical feet to the summit and was anchored to the side of the mountain with pickets. We then hooked onto the rope with mechanical ascenders that would greatly reduce the risk of falling off the steep slope.

It was a considerable thrill to be hanging off the side of a seemingly vertical incline miles above the huts and llamas in the valley below.

Before long, I was thinking in terms of larger mountains and more ambitious projects. One day while driving to work, the idea came to me. I knew exactly what I wanted to do, and I knew Peter would help make it happen. As soon as I got to the office, ignoring the blinking light on my answering machine, I called Summits Adventure Travel. When Peter answered, I outlined my vision.

"Peter, I just had an idea. I want to climb a bigger mountain, I'm ready for a bigger mountain, and I want to do it for breast cancer, with other survivors. It would send an incredible message about survival, will, and hope. What do you think?"

"Laura, I'm tiling the bathroom. Can I call you back later?" Peter replied.

"Later" was barely five minutes. Peter was intrigued by the idea and set his bathroom remodeling aside.

"Laura, I like the idea. Tell me more about what you have in mind."

We talked for a half hour that day, an hour the next. We agreed that the concept was a good one, but we debated which mountain would be the best .

I thought Mount McKinley made sense. Peter had a better idea.

"I know the perfect location. Aconcagua in Argentina. It's a beautiful mountain and one that outside of climbing circles people know very little about. It's higher than McKinley but not as logistically difficult. We would have a greater chance for success."

The decision was made. Aconcagua it would be. Two days later, Peter christened the climb "Expedition Inspiration," and we were off and running.

In those first weeks, as we put structure to our project and assembled a press packet, I remember Peter saying, "This will either be small or huge. It won't be in between. It will be one or the other." Either way seemed fine with me.

"I just want to see it happen," I informed Peter in one of our many ensuing conversations. "I want people to know that there can be life after breast cancer and that a positive attitude can make a difference. Women are so scared when they go through this disease, and they so often feel all alone. We can help educate and empower these women and make people aware of how little is being done to curb this epidemic."

But as committed as I was, I still spent an agonizing week soul-searching, reviewing what I was about to do. I had a little conversation with my inner self. *Now, Laura, are you sure this is what you want to do? Climbing is your solace, your escape, your release, the only time you are totally removed from everything else in the world. Do you want to take that public? Turn it into a possible media event? Just be clear in your mind about the repercussions of this project, and make certain it's what you really want.*

It was, I decided. I believed I was alive for a reason. I had almost died, but I hadn't. I had made a vow when first diagnosed that if I survived I would somehow help others who face this same crisis in their lives. I had a debt to repay, an obligation or perhaps a calling. I saw the positive reaction to my new direction from all the women in my wellness group and the overwhelming response to my climb up Kilimanjaro. An article had been written in the *Idaho Mountain Express* entitled "Active Wellness Propels Local Woman to the Top of Kilimanjaro." The day after the feature appeared, every copy of the paper in town had been picked up and the article cut out, tacked to bulletin boards, and sent to friends. Numerous people, including the mayor of Sun Valley, said that the message of "living your life now" had changed the way they would conduct their lives in the future. I knew we could touch many more lives with a climb up Aconcagua, the highest mountain in the world outside of the Himalayas.

And besides, once I was on the mountain, nothing would change, with or without cameras. It would still be me and the mountain, one on one. I would, as before, find myself lulled into a gentle space, separated from any outside influences. I would get caught up in the singular satisfying focus and repetitive rhythms of rest stepping and pressure breathing, and I would take others with me to experience it for themselves. There would be a lot of work between now and then, but once I was on the mountain, all would be okay.

It's interesting to me that people are often puzzled that I climb, that I love to climb. One friend recently inquired, "Why, when you came so close to death and got your life back, do you risk losing it climbing?"

I remembered a passage I had written in my diary:

When climbing, I am distanced from the day-to-day stresses of life. The quiet strength and beauty of the mountains nourish me, and I like the challenge of pitting myself against this incredible force of nature. Perhaps for one fleeting moment on the summit of a mountain, smiling into the camera lens, fists clenched and raised, I am invincible. I am immune to the disease that ravaged my body and soul, immune to all that I cannot control. I feel so in control, briefly, on top of the world. I believe, in doing that, I've gained some of the centuries-old strength from the mountain and it's now mine and nobody can ever take it from me.

Stated simply, whatever time I had left, I wanted it to be full of things I was passionate about. Mountaineering gave me a high, an energizing boost that I could not duplicate elsewhere. And, as with any major accomplishment, the sheer act of pushing myself to the limit made everything else easier. After you've climbed a peak, literally or figuratively, and you hear someone say, "Oh, the car's broken down, we're going to have to walk two miles in the cold," it's no big deal. Any sort of stress or problem is reduced after I've really tested myself physically and mentally. And I love the appreciation climbing gives me for my everyday life. Food, almost any food, tastes infinitely better after a week or two in the outback. My mattress is softer, my home warmer. How can one know hot without cold, soft without hard, pleasure without having endured pain?

Mountaineering is a most interesting activity. It is and it isn't a team sport. You climb as a group, conscious of one another's health and safety, often roped together over treacherous terrain, relying on your team members' knowledge and experience should someone fall. But you take every step alone, digging deep, focused on the goal and your own inner strength. Climbing, in many respects, is not unlike facing a life-threatening illness.

Soon after we started to promote Expedition Inspiration, people would ask me, "Why a mountain? Why climb a mountain for breast cancer?" I had a ready answer.

"In climbing a mountain and dealing with breast cancer, you face your deepest fear, the reality of death.

"You have to summon up all your strength physically and emotionally to reach your objective.

"Each is an individual struggle that is more effectively handled with team support.

"In order to survive, it takes one small courageous uphill step at a time.

"In the process, you find out what kind of person you are and what your ultimate values are. You develop a greater sense of self and self-worth."

As we continued to organize the Aconcagua climb, we realized that we needed an affiliation with a nonprofit agency to provide the third arm of a triangle. Peter would handle the logistics of the climb and be involved in much of the decision making. I would be responsible for selecting the team and managing the project. We also needed someone to help with fund-raising. We knew the project was unique enough to raise awareness, but we also wanted to raise a substantial amount of money for breast cancer research.

Neither Peter nor I had ever asked for a dime from anyone in our lives, so we were not at all sure where or how to begin finding a collaborator. But answers always come if you're looking.

One of the early applications we received was from Saskia Thiadens. She is the founder of the National Lymphedema Network in San Francisco and the nurse who had helped cure my lymphedema. I had never forgotten her magic or our hopeful conversations about how someday we would hike together. Saskia's early contribution to Expedition Inspiration was to introduce us to Andrea Martin, a two-time breast cancer survivor who quickly saw the merit in what we were doing. Andrea had recently started the Breast Cancer Fund in San Francisco, and she agreed to be a part of our project by using her organization to help fund-raise. She even set the ambitious goal of 2.3 million dollars, or one hundred dollars for each vertical foot of the mountain. Although two million dollars seemed like a lot of money, clearly it was only a fraction of what needed to be raised.

I had learned about the state of breast cancer research early on in my bout with the disease, and I had been shocked that so little was being done to find its causes. When I was diagnosed in 1989, 17 percent of all cancer deaths in the United States were breast cancer related, yet only 6 percent of the national funding was being allocated to any kind of breast cancer research. *What's wrong with this picture?* I remember thinking. *Why not an equal piece of the pie? How about 17 percent of the funding?* That was when I realized that breast cancer was low on the totem pole because it was a "woman's disease." What about wives and sisters, mothers, daughters, and the handful of men who get it themselves?

We were determined to call attention to a disease that had reached epidemic proportions and that was virtually being ignored. More money was desperately needed, and we wanted to figure out a way to raise it. Our first plan of action was to go to the Outdoor Retailer Trade Show in Reno. Both Peter Whittaker and I knew many people in the outdoor recreation industry, so, considering the nature of our project, it was a logical place to start.

We approached JanSport almost as soon as the doors to the show opened. Not only does JanSport, a leading manufacturer of packs, tents, and active sports apparel, dominate the industry in sales volume, it is a humanitarian company run by fun, caring people. Both Peter and I knew the president, Paul Delorey, well enough to feel comfortable approaching him with Expedition Inspiration.

I started. "Paul, we are planning an expedition in Argentina. It will be a fund-raiser for breast cancer and a vehicle to raise awareness and hope. I am a breast cancer survivor and, with Peter, will co-lead a team of other survivors up Aconcagua. We were hoping you would be interested in being one of our sponsors. We have a press kit outlining the project."

"Yes," Paul replied without hesitating.

Yes? Peter and I looked at each other. *It can't be this easy,* we were both thinking.

"Let me tell you a story," Paul began. "When I was a kid, I had an aunt who died, leaving behind four small children. When three of them, Mary, Pete, and Larry, came to live with us, it was hard for me to understand why their mother had died. It was nice to always have someone to play with, but it was a lot of work for my mother. I didn't realize until later that their mother, my aunt, had died of breast cancer. I never forgot that. I'd be happy to help."

Our efforts to generate support at the trade show snowballed from that moment on. Before long other outdoor equipment companies were trying to locate us instead of the other way around. Word was out that JanSport was the lead sponsor of a unique and exciting new climb, a climb for a cause. Although a recent climb up McKinley in support of AIDS had been backed by a few firms, the outdoor industry was typically pretty insular. It seemed there were always environmental and wildlife concerns, but this industry had not really ventured out into the larger arena. To support an expedition for breast cancer was unique. As we soon found out, even in the outdoor industry many lives had been touched by this horrific disease; it should not have come as a surprise.

The afternoon of our first day at the show, Peter and I were seated at a small round table crowded in among clothing samples in the back of one of the booths. Opposite us sat John and Neide Cooley, two of the principals of Marmot Mountain, Ltd.

Peter and I sat there stunned. We had only started recruiting supporters six hours earlier. Already we had secured commitments from the top manufacturers of outdoor sports gear. If only we could get Marmot, more critical pieces of our equipment list would be taken care of. But something was wrong.

Peter shifted his gaze away from Neide, who had been crying since we had arrived at their booth several minutes earlier. Her overwhelming grief was evident in her slumped shoulders, her lined brow. Finally, she spoke.

"It was my sister-in-law, last year. It was so unexpected," Neide said, trying to compose herself. "We are obviously very close to this subject. We very much want to be involved."

Another victim. My heart went out to Neide and to her sister-in-law. How many times had I heard this before? How easily this could have been David or Mike, my brothers-in-law, talking about me.

It was clear to us from the response at the trade show that Expedition Inspiration represented a combination of physical and spiritual strength, a climb people could look up to and maybe through which they could in some small way change the lives of those touched by breast cancer. Not until much later did I realize that picking a macho vehicle—a mountain climb—to call attention to breast cancer allowed men and women alike to feel comfortable talking about a "woman's" disease.

Companies like JanSport, Marmot, Salomon, Outdoor Research, Duofold, Moving Comfort, and Leki gave us everything we asked for, in each case a contribution larger than they had ever made in the past or ever thought they would make. Companies like Raichle set aside a portion of the proceeds from the products they sold to go toward breast cancer research. We also received free ad space and glowing editorials from almost every magazine connected with the outdoor industry. It was very heartening.

JanSport's public relations firm, GMR Marketing, hastily wrote and produced a very effective and emotionally packed promo video that kicked off our press conference. And JanSport's ad agency, Elgin Siefert DDB Needham, donated its time and talent to produce our first national ad. In it there is a likeness of a climber, presumably me, scaling an ice wall with the caption, "When diagnosed with breast cancer, women may go through many stages: Denial. Fear. Self-pity. Or in Laura Evans' case, the insatiable urge to kick ass." The ad was featured in most of the outdoor magazines and became a celebration of determination, of the will to fight back. The reaction was more favorable than we could have ever envisioned.

Comments flowed in daily. "I have the kick-ass ad tacked to the wall of my hospital room. It keeps me going." "If you can climb mountains, I can get through chemo." "If you can climb to 23,000 feet, I can start walking." The continuing stream of phone calls and letters made it easier to put in the long hours it took to coordinate the myriad details involved in a major climb and fund-raising effort. But, beyond that, I felt I was indeed one of the lucky ones. Not only was I alive, but my dream of helping others deal with crisis in their lives was coming true. There was no longer any question in my mind as to why I was alive. I was destined to show others, by example, that there is hope.

CHAPTER 16

The Response

Example is not the main thing in
influencing others. It is the only thing.

Albert Schweitzer

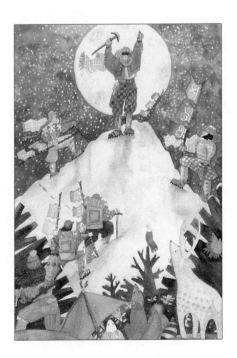

If I can give something back, if some good can come of my illness, then I will know that all this suffering has not been without purpose.

———————■———————

When you start a project, especially a large, highly visible one, you can never be certain how it will turn out or how it will be received. But the overwhelming reaction from the manufacturers and media in the outdoor industry confirmed that what we were doing was worthwhile. What we hadn't considered was that Expedition Inspiration would have a profound effect on how mountain-climbing expeditions would be viewed in the future.

One of the first articles about Expedition Inspiration was written by Joan Alvarez, the publisher and editor of *Outdoor Retailer* magazine. The piece was entitled "So What?" and explained why she, personally, was backing our project—in the form of seven free ads and many editorials. She wrote,

> *Almost every day it seems we hear from some outdoor-hearty soul looking for funds to underwrite his or her latest expedition. When determining whether or not to lend support to one of these endeavors, I ask myself several questions: What is the long-term social value of the undertaking? What difference will it make to the quality of life on this planet? What's the motivation behind it? What's the end goal?* Outdoor Retailer *is proud to have lent both financial and administrative support to several*

laudable expeditions over the years. This year we're espe-
cially pleased to offer our support to Expedition Inspira-
tion: Aconcagua, a 23,000-foot climb of the highest
mountain in the Western Hemisphere. Expedition Inspi-
ration clearly passes the "So What?" criteria and deserves
as much support as it can get.

Andrea Gabbard, who was the official Expedition Inspiration journalist, added, "The outdoor community being involved in an expedition like this is really important. It makes us blink and realize that there's a world beyond the vacuum we're used to working in, and demonstrates how much of a contribution we, as an industry, can make to the greater good of the world."

Peter and I were featured on the cover of *Sporting Goods Business,* and we were thrilled by the additional exposure and its potential for helping us achieve our goals. We hoped we would receive the same response from the general public that we were getting from the outdoor industry. We knew that many breast cancer survivors and supporters of the cause had never owned a backpack. We wanted them also to become more conscious of how many women and men were being affected by breast cancer and more aware of what was and wasn't being done. We also wanted to reach individuals to empower them with our message.

And we did.

Letters and phone calls poured in daily. Piles of articles and handwritten notes flowed into our office. One woman wrote, "I find it amazing that there are still people who understand life and know how to live it." Another woman, who was struggling with the disease, replied, "I guess each of us faces our own mountain. As I face the remainder of my treatment I will recall the inspiring article about your journey in the *Oregonian* newspaper and focus on the future." Yet another thanked us for "kicking her in the butt" and giving her the strength to get her life back together.

Timing, I know, is a big part of the success of any endeavor, and our timing was perfect. Coming off the excesses of the eighties, we as a nation were entering a period of social responsibility, of concern for our fellow human beings. With that, thank God, came an increased interest in our health and well-being and the feel-good stories that offered hope. The encouraging response to Expedition Inspiration from many parts of the world demonstrated the far-reaching effects that a project focusing on the positive can have.

The most surprising and interesting coverage was that of the *Yomiuri Shimbun* of Japan, the largest-circulation newspaper in the world. The writer was fascinated that women would try such a tough physical challenge and would also be so vocal about a disease that in their country patients are not even told they have. When I first heard this, it seemed inconceivable to me. Here we were, exerting all this time and effort to inform others by laying out everything we had been through, while in Japan doctors handed their patients a bottle of medicine without a word. I admitted, however, that I knew little about their society and recognized that social change took time. Because of the radical differences in approach to disease in our two countries, I was pleased with the *Yomiuri*'s response to what we were doing. They ultimately aided in our educational process. One article touched on, among other things, the positive benefits and possible healing qualities of outdoor activity for breast cancer survivors. The paper reported, "Dr. Michael Kelley, who with his colleagues has been researching the effect such activities as climbing might have on the immune system, postulates that the unusual combination of mental and physical activity needed to climb successfully creates a positive physical response."

Kelley went on to say that although there was no empirical or scientific data to support an association between climbing and recovery, he and some of his colleagues believed that there was a relationship between the outdoor adventure activities and changes in mental and neuroimmunological systems.

In addition to the *Yomiuri Shimbun*, articles followed in *Outside Magazine, Women's Sports and Fitness, Shape, Redbook, Self, Elle, Parade* magazine, *Business Week*, the *Chicago Tribune*, the *New York Times*, and many, many others.

Bylines saluted "the courageous team of breast cancer survivors who would face the second greatest challenge of their lives" and talked about "the ascent or upward movements of the spirit that at first are in tune then finally in opposition to the inevitable course of physical strength and health." In every article was the message that we were climbing "for our lives and those of others."

Expedition Inspiration snowballed—so much that my own health became an issue. It was wonderful to help others, but I would be useless if I were to get sick again. So I began to concentrate on working as hard as I could without overdoing it. But even on the long days, another letter or call would come in thanking us for what we were doing. The gratification of knowing that our gift was helping others made all the effort worthwhile. It was impossible to lose perspective on why we were doing the climb.

Still, I kept one of Goethe's sayings taped to my wall as another reminder of the thousands of women out there battling breast cancer:

> The world is so empty
> if one thinks only of
> mountains, rivers and cities:
> but to know someone here & there
> who thinks and feels with us,
> and who, though distant
> is close to us in spirit
> this makes the earth for us
> an Inhabited Garden.

CHAPTER 17

Shakedown Climb

Tough times don't last,
tough people do.

Summits' guides

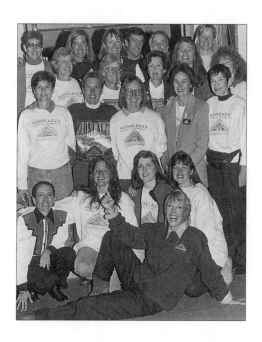

I love the natural wisdom, humility, and acceptance that come to those who spend time in the wilderness. In the mountains it is just you, stripped to the core, smelly, fearful, unsure about what lies ahead, with only your attitude and will to see you through. It is survival, learning to live with less and rely on others more.

———————————■———————————

I paced nervously in front of the Nisqually Lodge in Ashford, Washington, near the entrance to Rainier National Park. I had been waiting for this moment for over a year and, in some ways, all my life. I stretched my neck to try and see around the bend in the road that led back to Seattle, but my line of vision was obstructed by trees. I walked to the end of the curved driveway hoping for a better view, found none, and headed back to the entrance of the inn.

I thought about that morning. Most of my time had been spent sorting through the boxes JanSport had sent, boxes that contained Expedition Inspiration logo packs, T-shirts, mugs, hats, and sweaters. The team would be delighted. More stuff. If there ever was a real live Santa, it was Paul Delorey, JanSport's president. Not only had his company underwritten the total cost of the expedition, but he personally made sure we were adequately supplied with custom-embroidered clothing and gear.

The team. *Where are they?* I wondered as I continued to walk back and forth in front of the lodge. *They should have been here an hour ago.* I could barely contain my excitement. I felt like a mother hen. This was my team. I had selected each one carefully from hundreds of applications. Over the last months I had left encouraging messages on our 800-number line, sometimes daily. I had carefully ordered, packed, and shipped each person's equipment. I had met some of them personally but not all of them. Would they be as I imagined, so wonderfully full of life? This would be the first time we would all be together, in the flesh, women from such varied walks of life, from all over the country. Our one common bond was breast cancer and a desire to see something done about it.

I thought about my first meeting with Claudia Crosetti and Nancy Johnson from Ukiah, California. It had taken place nine months earlier, after several phone calls. We had agreed to meet in Sausalito, while I was in the Bay Area for my six-month checkup. I reached the restaurant we had designated a few minutes ahead of time. Claudia and Nancy were already there. Both of them popped out of their seats as I rounded the corner onto the patio.

"You must be Laura," they said in unison, smiling broadly. I could tell they were anxious and eager at the same time.

"This is my dad," Claudia remarked once we were seated. "He helps me work out. In fact, I bet he would like to go." She glanced at her dad, punctuating her comment with light nervous laughter. Claudia's dad reminded me of my dad, and I couldn't suppress a pang of sadness. I knew how proud my father would have been of Expedition Inspiration.

Claudia had an impish quality. Her eyes twinkled as she spoke, and her short dark hair bounced around on her head. I could tell she was fit, which she confirmed a moment later.

"We've been hiking up and down the hills in Ukiah," she explained, smiling at Nancy. "We even went out last week in the rain! People thought we were nuts.

"And Dad's helping motivate me," she added, patting her father on the arm. "So I know I can be in good enough shape." She took a breath and continued, "The chemo left me a little weak and off center. This climb would be a really positive experience and great incentive to get back into excellent shape physically and mentally."

Claudia was on a roll. "Nancy and I have also done a lot for the breast cancer cause in Ukiah and want to stay involved. It would be wonderful to have the opportunity to help out on a national level." Another smile for Nancy. "I was so excited when Kathleen Grant told me about Expedition Inspiration. She is the one who encouraged me to apply. I can't believe we have the same oncologist."

On that note, Claudia settled back in her chair, as if cuing Nancy to state her case.

Nancy had been so quiet I'd almost forgotten she was there. As I waited for her to speak, I got the distinct impression that she thought this was Claudia's deal. Even though she wanted to go, she didn't have much of a chance.

And she was partially right. I felt I had to decide between them. I wanted to round out the team with women from as many different states as possible. Two from the same California town probably didn't make sense. But, even though Nancy may not have realized it, the decision would be difficult, I knew, for I had carefully read both their résumés.

I watched Nancy as she spoke. With her close-cropped hair and lean build, she looked like a tomboy. "I made a conscious decision early on in my struggle with breast cancer not to allow this experience to fossilize into yet another silence," she began. I thought back to Nancy's résumé. There had been another illness years before, but in our phone conversations she had never talked about it. "Expedition Inspiration affords me the opportunity to share my passion to increase awareness, raise funds for research, and to offer hope. Everyone going through breast cancer has difficult days, and by being a part of this climb I would hope to give them strength to get through those tough times."

There was a restraint or a sadness about Nancy that I couldn't quite pinpoint, but there was also a sincerity that I felt could be an asset when lending support to others.

They detailed, once again, all they had done in their community to help educate others and to raise money to support other breast cancer patients. They also emphasized, again, their strong desire to be a part of our project and the commitment they would make to see it through. I knew a choice was impossible. I was seated in front of two energetic, personable women who embodied everything we were looking for in terms of spokeswomen and participants for the climb.

They were the first two team members selected to be a part of Expedition Inspiration.

Where is the team, anyway? The bus should have been here long ago. As I continued my vigil, I thought about Kim O'Meara Anderson, the thirty-five-year-old mother and runner from Iowa. Her application had torn at my heartstrings. "Diagnosed while breast-feeding my first and only child." And her comment on the phone, "I really want to help with the breast cancer cause. I've called many organizations to tell them I want to help out, but they always tell me I'm geographically undesirable because of where I live. They say they would let me help if I lived on one of the coasts." For Expedition Inspiration, she was geographically desirable, our first Midwesterner. We met in a hotel coffee shop, and I was immediately endeared to her humility and conviction.

My thoughts were interrupted when I caught sight of a van rounding the corner and heading up the drive. I waved my arms in greeting, smiling broadly, aware of the laughter and good feelings emanating from the bus. *It obviously didn't take long for this team to bond,* I observed.

I greeted each of my team members with a hug, not needing to be reminded who was who, calling up mental notes of each woman's story. *No surprises,* I thought, *a great group of women.*

After everyone found her room, the new gear was distributed. Excited laughter and endless hugs filled the afternoon. I was reminded of a sign in my office that reads, "No one ever died from an overdose of hugs." I give and receive hugs as often as possible. All that time in isolation in the hospital only increased my need for hugs. The embraces that afternoon, I sensed, were the beginning of a closeness and a sharing that would intertwine the lives of these people for a long time to come. They would ensure that the goodwill and collective passion for the mission of Expedition Inspiration would spread far beyond this group.

That night we piled into the van for the five-mile drive to the Gateway Inn, the rustic log restaurant and gift shop where we would have our first meal together. Joining us were our team doctors, guides, and a couple of sponsors—in all, more than thirty people. We descended on the restaurant en masse, pouring into the back room. We filled the lengths of many tables that had been configured into a T, then we overflowed into the booths bordering two sides of it.

It took a while to get everyone seated, since the energy and elation in the room were almost too great to harness. In the back of everyone's mind was the fact that the following day we would begin our climb up the most treacherous mountain in the continental United States. This would be our prelim to Aconcagua. For most of the team, this was a new adventure. That anticipation was compounded by the interest we had in one another. We were united by a common pledge, but we were still strangers, unfamiliar, as of yet, to the nuances that made each of us individuals. It was important to get to know one another and to start thinking like a team.

Peter Whittaker planned to give a brief orientation to make everyone aware of what to expect over the next few days, but first we went around the room to hear from each person more about why she was here.

I began. "Most of you know my story, probably by heart by now, so I won't repeat it. I will only say that I am extremely grateful to be alive and to be here in this room with all of you. I don't think I can adequately describe how happy I am to have us all here together, to see those of you again whom I met briefly and to meet those of you I had not met but feel that I already know. I want to welcome you and thank you for being a part of Expedition Inspiration and for your dedication to the breast cancer cause. With our combined enthusiasm, we can help a lot of women and can raise the money and awareness to help put an end to this horrible disease. We will talk more later in the weekend about fund-raising, but for now I think it is important for us to get to know one another. Why don't we start at the end of the table and have each of you stand up and tell us a little about what you have been through?"

Roberta Fama began. "When I was diagnosed, all of my girlfriends were having babies while I was facing a modified radical mastectomy and six months of chemo."

Roberta was from the San Francisco area and had struggled with breast cancer for years. She was also one of our youngest team members. The room grew quiet as she continued, "The doctors didn't tell me that because of the treatment I would never be able to get pregnant," she recited, unable to hold back the tears. Kim, seated next to her, took her hand. "I was only twenty-eight," Roberta added. "Not only did cancer cost me my children, but there was a pretty good chance that it would cost me my life as well." She hesitated before going on. "Two years after the mastectomy, I had back surgery because it had spread to my spine, but I want people to know that even if cancer comes back, it doesn't have to be the beginning of an end. I'm still alive and I thank God each day that I'm happy and healthy and hope that through this project I can give something back."

I could see the love and support in the faces of the other survivors. Yes, I know. Yes, I've been there. Yes, I'm so sorry.

Patty Duke was next. "Hi, I'm Patty Duke!"

"The real Patty Duke?" someone hollered.

"Well, no, not the real Patty Duke," she grinned. Patty was adorable. She hailed from Steamboat, Colorado, and had recently started a sock company catering to outdoor sports enthusiasts. With Patty's pretty face and shoulder-length flip, she didn't look like she had been sick a day in her life. But when she talked about cancer and her young boys, tears welled in her eyes. "I had three types of cancer: tubular, lobular, and ductal. I found a lump in my breast, but it wasn't a little lump. It spread from my chest all the way under my arm," she said as her hand swept across the front of her body. "One day my son came up to me and said, 'Mom, are you going to die?'" Patty balanced herself with one hand on the side of the table and looked around the room. "Because of what I have been through, I have found that there are things that mean a lot more than before and there are things that don't mean so much anymore. Surprisingly, life is better. I want to do this climb to show other women that they can climb through anything."

"Yeah, right on," another survivor added, reinforcing Patty's sentiment.

Sara Hildebrand stood up. Sara, from Neenah, Wisconsin, was our oldest team member and adamant about educating women, especially those in her age group.

"Seventy percent of the two million women who have breast cancer and the one million who have it but don't know they have it are over sixty. But these women don't want to know if they have it. They won't go get a mammogram. Those are the women I'm climbing for. I want them to know that if cancer is detected early, it is not a death sentence."

Sue Anne Foster, a mother from Sacramento, California, talked about facing her fears and working through them. "I didn't want to be afraid. No matter if I lost my hair or had this terrible disease, I was still me. The whole emphasis and focus changed from fear of the future to living in the present and cherishing each moment."

Everyone listened intently, pooling our collective thoughts for later use in promoting the project.

Vicki Boriack was next. I had met Vicki at the outdoor show in Reno. She was working for a company called Mont Bell and had recently undergone one of her many chemotherapy treatments. She looked a lot better now. In fact, with her straight brown hair and freckled baby face, she looked ten years younger than her forty years. "I was diagnosed at the young age of thirty-nine and had a mastectomy," she began. "My husband had a hard time with my diagnosis and the fact that I had only one breast. I know cancer cost me my marriage. But my two kids have given me strength." I could see nods of agreement from Patty and Kim. Vicki paused for a moment before continuing, "If there's anything I've learned from a cancer diagnosis, it's that there is no time to waste. I'm going for it."

"Yes!" came an immediate response from several of the team members.

Nancy Hudson uncoiled her lanky five-foot-nine-inch frame and stretched up to her full height. "I wasn't even sure I wanted to do this. Laura practically had to talk me into it," she proceeded, looking my way. "I have two young sons and I teach art and I'm trying to get a divorce. I didn't think I could really get away for this long. I know I drove Laura nuts trying to make up my mind, but I'm really glad I'm here, with all of you," she added, looking around the table at her fellow survivors. She did almost drive me nuts. Nancy has enough energy for five or six people but some difficulty in harnessing it. I hoped this project would help her do just that.

"I was diagnosed with intraductal carcinoma of the left breast," Nancy was saying. "I had a mastectomy and twenty-five negative lymph nodes removed. I know I'm strong and can do this and that I can raise lots of money, which is probably why Laura put me on," she chuckled. "Also this climbing expedition would be another contribution I can make to my fellow survivors, as well as to myself, in our fight for breast cancer prevention."

"Okay, Nance, that's enough," someone said humorously, when Nancy started to ramble.

Sitting beside Nancy was Eleanor Davis, a soft-spoken, intelligent woman who was also our longest survivor. I had spoken with her several times on the phone. She had done a great deal over the years to help other women with breast cancer and to raise funds for research. She was also a former pilot who trekked all over the world. I felt she was a great addition to the team. "I'm from Pennsylvania," she began, "and I had bilateral mastectomies twelve years ago. You didn't talk about breast cancer back then. You just dealt with it and got on with your life.

"Since I was diagnosed, I have been a volunteer for the American Cancer Society, helping others deal with this disease. But Expedition Inspiration has really given me the opportunity to deal personally with my experience with breast cancer and to talk openly about my feelings. This project also allows me to represent and bring hope to all women who have breast cancer."

Several women clapped.

Annette Porter, from Seattle, was the sexiest of our team members. As she talked about her struggle with going bald, she unselfconsciously stroked her luxurious ten-inch mane of hair. "That was the hardest part for me. I didn't look sick or feel sick until I lost all my hair, and it was hard for me to deal with. I'm a photographer, and I started taking pictures of myself and other women with no hair to show that it was all right, part of the process. Photographing other women helped me deal with my loss. It was letting go of the things I couldn't control."

Most women in the room had lost their hair, so we all knew what it felt like.

"I never thought I'd do either one," Annette contemplated, "be a part of a mountain-climbing expedition or fight breast cancer. But having done the latter, I couldn't imagine not doing the former. Both are celebrations of life, empowering and humbling at the same time. With cancer, as with climbing, I find you need a huge support group to get through it."

"You have that support group now," Nancy mentioned, and everyone nodded in agreement.

Claudia Berryman-Shafer, from Fernley, Nevada, looked every bit like the long-distance runner she was. Her powerful legs were about twice the size of anyone else's. Although she was still undergoing chemo, no one would ever know. "The week after surgery, I went out and ran ten miles until my doctor told me to slow down," she recalled, her face lighting up with an impish grin. "I really look at Expedition Inspiration as an opportunity to put cancer behind me. I am not interested in dealing with it anymore. I want to move forward."

By the time the last team member had spoken, there was not a sound in the room except for an occasional nose being blown. For us, the survivors, this in a way was old hat. We had heard the stories before. We knew, intimately, the pain, fear, and discomfort that each of us had just described, but now we were a team, a family, and the stories were those of women who were now connected to our lives. We knew we were giving courage to others by doing something that most people wouldn't dream of doing. We were united but saddened by how much we had all suffered, knowing all too well how many other women were suffering the same things. But we were also uplifted by how we had all survived and the spirit we all showed.

Each woman's story was compelling, but to hear them told in the first person, one after another, in the darkened back room of that cozy inn sent chills up everyone's spines. These were survivors. These were women who had looked into the gaping jaws of death and dug in their heels, summoning up every ounce of strength they possessed to stay alive.

For the guides and sponsors, the trauma and determination of what they had just witnessed was an eye opener. Here was a group of women who looked fit and healthy, totally belying the reality of the devastating, life-threatening disease that we had all faced.

The silence lengthened until finally John Cooley, the president and CEO of Marmot, stood up. "I am extremely proud to be a part of this group," he began, trying to compose himself in the process. "I have done a lot of climbing. In the early years, people always talked about the brotherhood of the rope. In the eighties and nineties more women started climbing, and we talked about the sisterhood of the rope. But with Expedition Inspiration, we have moved to another level, and that is the humanness of the rope. It is not about the ego gratification of getting to the top of the mountain; it is about helping others on the way."

We had never thought of it in exactly those terms. We all listened intently.

"I know the strength it takes to get to the summit, but I am humbled by the stories I have heard here tonight. I feel as if I am on the other side of a door, unable to really appreciate what you have been through. It is hard to fathom the incredible willpower and determination it has taken for you to reach the summit that each of you has reached just by being here today. I would like to propose a toast to the women of Expedition Inspiration."

Everyone raised her glass in a teary-eyed salute.

"I would also like to make a toast," spoke Kate Casson, one of the guides. "I have been guiding on Rainier for ten years and I've met a lot of strong people, but I've never met anyone like you guys. You can teach me and others what strength really is."

I had known Kate for many years through my trips to Rainier. She is a little bitty woman with a shock of red hair, but her looks are no indication of her strength. I had often seen her carry her own body weight in gear on her back and had always considered her one of the physically strongest women I knew.

The women in this room were tough. I used to have a saying taped to my phone that read, "You are only as tough as what you have suffered." These women had all garnered strength from their bout with cancer and the emotional process of getting through it. They were physically fit and mentally prepared for the challenges that lay ahead. I knew and the guides knew that we had a formidable team here. Not everyone might reach her goal, but each would give it her all, enduring whatever hardships came her way.

I was reminded of a letter that had been sent to the team containing these words of wisdom: "A word on focus. There are two summits on a mountain. The physical summit and one's own personal summit. If you have the energy, you can reach the physical summit; however, the most difficult summit to reach is your personal limit." This would be proven out on Mount Rainier over the next few days.

Most of the team members had never climbed before, and for that reason they were assigned to the trek team, "the heart of the team," in the words of my oncologist, Dr. Kathy Grant. The trekkers would ascend to Mount Rainier's Nisqually Glacier, several hours below Camp Muir at 10,000 feet. At Nisqually they would set up camp, then advance to Muir the following day. The "body of the team, " or the summit team, would climb to Muir, rest for a few hours, then embark for the summit, leaving in the early morning hours. If all went well, the two teams would meet the next day at 10,000 feet, as the trek team came up from Nisqually and we were descending from the summit.

Peter made it clear that although this was a shakedown climb, we were still a team. "If you don't make it to the summit or to Muir, that doesn't mean you're off the team. This is going to give you an idea of how tough it's going to be in Argentina. Aconcagua is a big mountain. Look at this weekend as an opportunity to see if your training is working or if you need to step up the pace."

The morning after our first dinner, we assembled in the parking lot at the Paradise Lodge. It was one of the most beautiful days in memory, the sky an intense shade of sapphire, uninterrupted by clouds. We were dressed in T-shirts and shorts, and we lathered on the sunscreen, thanking the weather gods. Above us, Rainier glistened, beautifully etched against the vast backdrop of blue.

Word was out that breast cancer survivors were going to climb the mountain, and many well-wishers, along with newscasters from Seattle television and radio stations, mingled in the glow of that obviously magical day. We heard later about two women who didn't arrive in time to send us off but who had heard about the project and wanted to meet us. Their niece had just been diagnosed with breast cancer, and they wanted to hike up Rainier as far as they could in her honor and in support of what we were doing. Hearing that story only reinforced in our minds why we were there.

I had climbed Rainier many times but always for the sole satisfaction of climbing. Although the mountaineering itself never gets easier, on this trip I was buoyed by the mission of Expedition Inspiration and the camaraderie of my team, my sister soul mates. I took great pleasure in seeing them revel in the beauty and challenge of this majestic element of the great outdoors.

The summit team at that time consisted of myself, Claudia Berryman-Shafer, Annette Porter, and Vicki Boriack, all of whom had had breast cancer. Paul Delorey of JanSport, Saskia Thiadens and Bud Alpert, our medics, James Kay, photographer, Andrea Gabbard, journalist, and Peter Whittaker, our fearless leader, as well as additional guides completed the team. Later we added two more survivors, Nancy Knoble from Tiburon, California, and Mary Yeo of Cumberland, Maine, to the summit team and Ashley Sumner-Cox to the trek team.

Of the summit team members, Vicki and Claudia were the two trying to climb while still undergoing chemo. A remarkable feat, to say the least, since most people are so weakened by the treatment that merely walking can often be a chore.

Several members of the trek team felt they were strong enough to be on the summit team and would have liked the opportunity to try. But climbing to higher altitudes appears easier before you experience what goes on up there. For safety reasons, we limited the summit team to those who had previously been at high altitude. Ultimately, we were a team, and everyone was pleased to be a part of it.

When we prepared to start the summit climb, the trek team saw us off amid a great deal of emotion.

"You come back safely, you hear?" Roberta told Vicki as she held her in a bear hug.

"You be careful, you guys," added Nancy Hudson.

"You take care of everybody," Erika reflexively instructed Peter.

And we were off, turning around only two or three times to get a last glimpse of the waving arms and smiling faces of the trekkers.

Because of the ideal weather conditions, we kept an easy pace, stopping three or four times before reaching Pebble Creek. Shortly thereafter Vicki was forced to turn. She knew going in how debilitated she felt from her last dose of chemo, but she still hoped she could at least make it to Muir. We were all disappointed—for her and for the team.

"It's okay, Vicki," we told her, trying to provide what comfort we could.

"I could never have made it this far while I was undergoing chemo," I pointed out.

But Vicki was disappointed. She wanted to be with the team and to prove herself. Plus, she was looking forward to climbing Rainier, which she hadn't done before.

Sadly, we said our good-byes to Vicki as she headed down and we headed up.

We reached base camp tired but, oh, so pleased with the weather. Andrea was one of the only other team members, aside from me, who had been on Rainier before, and due to weather conditions she had been denied the summit many times. As Peter and Lou say, "When the mountain says no, it's no." You can never be sure what Mother Nature will dish up in the way of weather. On a subsequent trip up this very same mountain with my sister Lisa, it poured buckets, a bone-drenching, go-sit-by-the-fire rain. We made it less than a quarter of the way up the mountain before turning back, and we spent days drying out our gear.

The glorious weather we experienced on the shakedown climb was as good as it gets. That afternoon after our trek to Muir, we started to set up the tents, spaced fairly close together, on what reasonably flat spots we could find.

"Which pole goes where?" Saskia asked, perplexed.

"They are color coded," Claudia pointed out. "The silver ones go in the silver sleeves, the blue in the blue. . . ." Claudia was a third-grade teacher and very good at instructing people.

It took two people per tent to bend the poles and stretch the fabric to the point where the tip of each pole would fit snugly into the designated grommet. After the tents were assembled, we pounded our poles into the snow, securing the flys that had been draped over the top. As soon as the tents were ready, we began unloading our packs.

It was important to get our sleeping bags unrolled and our shelters up in the event the weather suddenly changed. It was also a good idea to get out of our sweaty shirts and into something warm and dry.

While we fiddled with our gear, Peter dug a three-foot-deep, six-foot-square snow pit that would be our kitchen. Water was quickly put on to boil. With the summit attempt scheduled for that night, it would be an early evening. By the time everything was set up, it was dark. Bundled in our down jackets, we ate second and third helpings of noodles mixed with tuna, loading up on fuel for the next day.

After a few "sleep tights" and a collective prayer that the next day would be clear, we turned in. It was around 8:00 P.M., allowing us six hours of rest before Peter would roust us for the summit attempt.

We were two to a tent, and Saskia was my tentmate.

"What are you going to do with your boots?" Saskia asked.

"I'm going to bring them inside," I responded. "I don't want to leave anything out that I need to put on right away. It's going to be dark and cold when we get up."

"What about your clothes?"

"Everything in the sleeping bag that I'll be wearing. And keep your water and headlamp handy."

Very early the next morning, I could hear the guides rustling around, beginning preparations for a light breakfast. I immediately wrestled myself out of my sleeping bag. I knew how quickly the time would pass before we would start to rope up and be on our way. I began to layer up for the climb—long underwear, fleece pants and top, and my heavy down parka, which would be stuffed into my pack alongside my rain gear once we began to move.

No one says much when awakened at 2:00 A.M. in the pitch dark on the side of a glacier. Everyone is lost in his or her own thoughts: *What will it be like? How will I do? Am I ready? Am I even awake?* I thought about previous trips up this formidable mountain. I remembered my first and only black eye, a souvenir from the rock slide that somehow put a vice grip on my boot, causing me to do a face plant. And I grimaced, thinking about the sled ride down with my broken ankle.

But that night some higher power was with us. The stars glistened with the promise of another clear, sunny day, and we all rose, rested and, as the saying goes, ready. Soon we were moving, spiraling up the mountain, a chain of lights bobbing gently in the darkness.

As we crested the rock fall at 12,000 feet, the sun poked through a blanket of clouds below us and backlit Little Tahoma, the wedge-shaped peak to the east. It was in the shadow of this awe-inspiring sight that we took our first break of the day. We stopped long enough for a much-needed drink of water, a bite to eat, a clothing adjustment, and, for some of us, a bathroom break.

Ahead was a section of the mountain known as Disappointment Cleaver. The name says it all. We were reminded by the guides that climbers had been left in sleeping bags, strapped to the side of the mountain, just below or just above the Cleaver, because they ran out of steam. This was a very disquieting thought.

The Cleaver is ruthless. Ask anyone who's been there. It is straight up with no place to stop. For the average climber that spells an hour of peak (no pun intended) exertion. Often you can reach out your hand and touch the ice wall in front of you without bending at the waist at all. Even though you are roped together, with crampons on your boots and an ice ax in your hand, one slip on this treacherous section of the climb, and you could end up speeding toward the maze of crevasses below, trailing the rest of your rope team behind you.

Saskia made the mistake of dwelling on this possibility and was glancing down often to see where she might land. By the time she reached the top of the small, welcome plateau of level ground where the rest of the team was waiting, she and Katie, her rope team guide, were ready to call it quits.

Disappointment Cleaver is scary, especially if you think about it too much or too long. Then the fear can become paralyzing. Fear is the most debilitating emotion, whether on a mountain or in any aspect of life, which is why I try so hard to confront it. I have been on mountains where I've dared to glance down at slick, white, slidelike surfaces or into the deep, frigid darkness of gaping crevasses. And I have momentarily caught my breath, knowing that one false move, one lapse in concentration, could end my adventure in a most unpleasant manner. And then I move on, cautiously, forcing my mind to think only of the incredible view that awaits me at the summit.

"I feel all right," Saskia was saying. "I don't know why, I just feel tired. I don't want to let you down," she wanted me to know.

"Saskia, it's okay. You made it this far; you did great." I was thinking that it was sad to see Saskia have to turn, but this was the purpose of a shakedown climb. It was far better to know now, here on Rainier at 13,000 feet, that someone was going to have a problem, than in Argentina, miles from civilization and at much higher altitudes.

We said good-bye to Saskia and continued up, traversing endless snowfields. Annette was in front of me, directly behind Peter. I could tell she was a quick learner. I could hear the distinctive whistle of her pressure breathing and noted that she had perfected her rest step.

"It's ideal being between you and Peter," she commented later. "I just follow his steps and your breathing." These basic but essential techniques would serve Annette well here and on Aconcagua.

Our last rest break brought us within a half hour of the summit. The remaining team members felt strong and would clearly make it. We sat there, so close to the top, looking high above Little Tahoma at Mount Baker, Mount Hood, and the flattened top of Mount Saint Helens. It was a glorious few minutes. The fact that we had been blessed with incredible weather was not lost on anyone, and it gave positive reinforcement to the special nature, the powerful message of our project, Expedition Inspiration.

The relatively short distance to the summit took longer than anticipated. Each step was followed by one more, then another, as if this last segment of the mountain had been put on a treadmill that kept repeating under our feet. But soon we reached the crater rim, which called forth broad smiles, hugs, kisses, and high-fives. We were elated, all of us thinking the same thought: that we were successfully on our way to Aconcagua.

Any point on the crater rim is considered the summit, even if it isn't the highest point on the mountain, but a few of us traversed the crater to the opposite side to sign the park service book that records the names and dates of those who make it. We then made our way up the short distance to the tippy top, the highest point on Mount Rainier. There we took our hero shots and Peter showed me where one day he would place my ashes. We all hugged one another and thanked the universe for this wonderful life.

Soon we started down, anxious to share our success with the rest of the team.

We had tried several times to make contact with the trek team via our two-way radios but had never been able to get through. We wanted our teammates to know that we were safe and destined to stand on the summit of Aconcagua. Going down, we made good time. Without mishap, we reached the rock fall and the last part of the descent that would take us into camp, reuniting us with the rest of our team. Just as we started down the rock slide, we heard a chorus of voices from the rock outcropping situated just above camp.

"YEAHHHH!"

We stopped and smiled. Across the wide snowfield, 1,500 feet away, we could just make out the specks that were our teammates, perched among the rocks.

"Quick, all together, we have to respond," Peter commanded, rounding us up with a sweeping motion of his arm.

"YEAHHHH!" we shot back.

"YEAHHHH!" came back at us again, like an echo bouncing off the walls of a deserted canyon.

The remaining distance between us and camp, between us and the animated, caring voices that were welcoming us home, slipped beneath our feet barely noticed. By the time we reached base camp, most of our team members were waiting with open arms and a huge juicy watermelon that the "heart of our team" had lugged up to 10,000 feet. In the glow of that first victory celebration, all thoughts of what we had been through on this climb and before vanished as quickly as the slices of fruit that we hastily devoured.

Life was, indeed, good. We were most definitely a team.

CHAPTER 18

Aconcagua

The purpose of life, after all, is to live it, to taste experience to the utmost, to reach out eagerly and without fear for newer and richer experience.

Eleanor Roosevelt

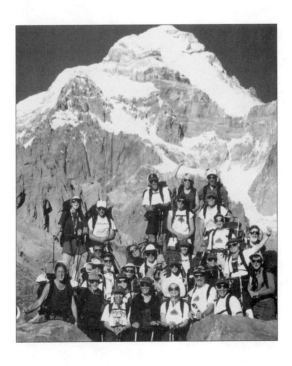

I reminisced today on the number of times in the hospital that I dreamed of climbing big mountains—purely a fantasy, like winning the lottery. I never really thought then that I would be here now, looking at this phenomenal mountain. It's impossible not to reflect on the gift of being alive in this beautiful wilderness, and it's hard not to cry in remembrance of the many, many women for whom we are climbing.

———————■———————

When the wheels of the plane left the ground and lifted as if weightless into the sky, the burden that had rested on my shoulders for so many months also lifted up and away, and I let out a huge sigh of relief.

Expedition Inspiration had become my life, the focal point of all my waking hours. In the last few months before the climb, my mind mulled over all the details. *What have I overlooked? Does everyone have all the gear she needs? What more needs to be done? Will the team members stay healthy, free from the dreaded cancer recurrence? Will I stay healthy? Will I make the summit of Aconcagua, as I am expected to? This will be the highest mountain I have ever climbed. And what's next? I have to work, but I don't want to go back to designing. That seems less important after what we have already achieved with this project. What will I do?*

All those thoughts drifted away as the wheels retracted into the fuselage of the plane and we rose higher, closer to Aconcagua.

The preparation was done now. From here on, we would be relying on our individual strength, buoyed by the support of our teammates. The mountain beckoned. The seemingly endless amounts of paperwork and phone calls for the project were no longer a part of my life, at least not for the next three weeks.

I relaxed into my seat and thought about the climb ahead. I thought about the Chinese symbol for crisis and its second meaning: "a dangerous opportunity." Yes, I had to agree. So often I hear women say that cancer changed their lives for the better, and I thought about all that had happened over the last two years. If I hadn't gotten cancer, I wouldn't have been on that plane headed to Argentina with sixteen incredible women, enjoying the personally rewarding response to a project that captured the imagination of thousands of people worldwide.

I'm glad that I can't reverse history, I thought. *I'm glad that I am unable to go back and change things, that I don't have to answer the question, If you had it to do all over again. . . .*

Sure, I wished I didn't have a pin and a screw in my ankle and that I hadn't once torn my hamstring and broken my knee. Yes, I wished often that I hadn't been thrown into early menopause and that I didn't almost wet my pants several times a day and that my stomach didn't rebel when I drank apple juice too fast. But no, I didn't want to change my life, where I was right then—as happy, fulfilled, and proud as I've ever been. Who knows where I would have been if things had been different?

I knew because of all the discomfort I had been through that I had increased my ability to push through pain and adversity in order to achieve a goal. I was hardier and was thankful for that. But I also knew that my resolve would be tested in the weeks to come. I just didn't realize how soon.

Of course I knew better, but I forgot for a moment that we were on a foreign carrier, and I brushed my teeth on the plane. I didn't notice the sign above the sink until I was rinsing my toothbrush. "Not drinking water." *Shit.*

By the time we arrived in Argentina, I was sick, plagued with serious diarrhea. Two days later I was throwing up, my stomach clenched into a ball because of cramps. *Oh, God. After all the time and effort and buildup, am I not going to make it to the summit of Aconcagua because I brushed my teeth on the plane?* I sought the advice of our team doctor, Bud Alpert, who put me on antibiotics, salt tabs, and as much water as I could force down.

Little by little I recovered, making myself drink and eat to ward off dehydration and to rebuild my strength. I would not let this get in my way.

I needed to stand on this summit for me, for the team, and for all the people who knew in their hearts that I would. Expedition Inspiration was like a fairy tale, where you already know or at least hope that it has a happy ending. Many people's faith in good things would have been shaken if on the last page the big bad wolf had eaten Goldilocks or if Laura Evans hadn't made the summit. I had made a pact with myself and everyone who had come into contact with Expedition Inspiration. I would stand on that summit.

I thought about the women on the team and how happy, healthy, and excited they were to be a part of this worthwhile adventure. Looking at our team, the average person would never know the fear, pain, and soul-searching that these women had gone through. Just a few faces in a crowd, we were like the millions of women who walk quietly with their secret burden of breast cancer and the unexpressed upheaval it has caused in their lives. We were only a handful, but our steps up Aconcagua would mirror those of many others in our collective search for answers to this devastating disease.

On January 22, after two nights in the Andean city of Mendoza, we boarded a bus bound for Puente del Inca, situated at

9,000 feet. Miles of rolling hills and a meandering muddy river provided the gateway to this mecca. The inn, hot springs, church, and conglomeration of hutlike souvenir stands that made up Puente del Inca would be the last civilized outpost before we hit the trail.

As we rolled through the arid environment, it was hard to imagine the wind, snow, and cold that awaited us at higher elevations. I looked out the window of the bus and recalled one of the guides' earlier comments, "Aconcagua is a tough mountain because it can lull you to sleep." I was certain that the colorfully painted hills I now viewed would soon enough be replaced with something altogether different.

As we neared Puente del Inca, Peter joked, "This inn won't look like much now, but it will look like a four-star hotel when we get off the mountain." He was right on both counts. Our final civilized accommodations were rustic. Long, narrow rooms were lined with bunk beds, and they shared an indoor outhouse down the hall. The food was as basic as the rooms, but it didn't really matter. We had other things on our minds.

The first day after arriving at Puente del Inca was spent acclimating to the 7,000-foot elevation, going through our gear and ditching what we didn't absolutely need. Because of the generosity of our sponsors, all of us had more than we were ultimately able to carry on our backs. We would have mules to transport our equipment to base camp at 13,800 feet, but from there on up we would be the beasts of burden. It was incredible to me how much gear a team of seventeen would need: 3,850 pounds. For the first part of the climb, this would be distributed among twenty-five or thirty mules that were provided and led by local muleteers. Each mule would carry up to 160 pounds.

The trek team would arrive a week later and would have its own mules and muleteers. My husband would be with them as one of the few men who would support the team. His encouragement, understanding, and support throughout the two long years of organizing the Aconcagua climb easily justified his participation. Besides, as the founder of Expedition Inspiration, I wanted him to share in the experience. The goal of the trek team would be to reach base camp at 13,800 feet. It would have been nice, but impractical, for the two teams to start the trip together. No one wants to spend more time than necessary on a mountain climb, so the time lapse would allow the summit team the extra days needed to acclimate, carry loads up the upper mountain, and hopefully arrive back at Camp One a day or two after the trek team reached base camp.

We were constantly being reminded of the challenge that lay ahead. That first night, three climbers came down from the mountain, racked with coughs, faces red and blistered from the sun and wind. Their eyes spoke of anguish, like those of refugees who have seen too much, longing for the comforts of an easier life. Reports of thigh-deep snow filtered down from other climbers. Only three or four climbers had made the summit in the last three weeks, which made us all acutely aware that, as our promotional poster said, "This is no walk in the park."

The lighthearted chatter on the bus ride up was now replaced with a quiet uneasiness. I was sure I was not the only one who thought about the T-shirt-and-shorts weather on Mount Rainier for our shakedown climb.

The project had been blessed so far. We hoped that we would be blessed with a weather window here as well. We all said our personal prayers.

The following day the sun came out and with it our optimism. As we wandered around the low-lying mountains that framed Puente del Inca, we chose, as my husband, Roger, had worded it, to be "blissfully ignorant" of what was transpiring 10,000 feet above us. The day was spent hiking up the Horcones River Valley, which was lined with breathtaking hills painted in layers of ochre, rust, charcoal, off-white, and green. Verdant valleys fell off in all directions. That acclimation hike would afford us our first look at Aconcagua. At the end of a long valley, the mountain loomed, a solid mass of rock and ice, beckoning. The first glimpse of our intended goal jump-started my nervous system, revving me up for the challenge. I forgot about the stomach cramps and nonstop diarrhea. This was our much-anticipated goal. The mountain was massive and, in its entirety, intimidating. But I knew we would tackle it in segments, one step at a time, until hopefully we would stand, spent but elated, on the top. Everyone shared the same excitement and awe. The next day we would be under way. We all knew how excited our trek team members must be—only a couple of days away from starting their trip.

At 9:15 A.M. on January 24, we prepared to head up the mountain. The long-awaited journey was about to begin. We boarded a bus to the trailhead.

"We're on our way!" Peter exclaimed. "How do you feel?"

"Great!"

"Fabulous!"

"Where are we going?" he asked.

"To the top!" Three or four of us responded at once.

With the first steps toward our goal, I felt very peaceful. We were on our way. What happened now was out of my hands. I thought about the first walk I had taken out of the hospital, devoid of strength. It was so different now as my body comfortably relaxed into the cadence of an accustomed stride.

It was a hot day, close to 85 degrees. The cloudless sky provided no barrier of protection against the intensity of the sun's rays, and layers of sunblock were our only hope. We remembered the climbers who had come down while we were at Puente del Inca. Many of their faces and arms had been red and raw from the ravages of sunburn. We tried to look out for each other.

"Hey, Nancy, did you put sunblock on your shoulders?" I inquired on one of our breaks.

"Yes. You probably need to put more behind your ears."

The trail meandered up and down a narrow valley, following the Las Vacas River. Occasionally strong gusts of wind would kick up grit, depositing it in our clothing, hair, and teeth. Regardless, the scenery was spectacular. Our route extended as far as the eye could see and was framed on two sides by 4,000 feet of jagged rock towering above us. It was too easy to revel in the views, forgetting to watch our footing, tripping on the colorful array of rocks that littered the trail. Ever vigilant, Peter would notice.

"Climb with your eyes, you guys," he would direct our way, as we maintained a steady pace. "One slip and you'll end up down there in the river."

We arrived in camp ahead of the muleteers. Unable to set up camp without our gear, four of us took our hot, dusty bodies down to the river. Finding a secluded spot with a quiet eddy, we disrobed and began to clean off the embedded grime.

"I feel so decadent," I commented, lifting my toes out of the water so that I could get to my feet. "Bare-ass naked in the wilderness."

Both Annette and Nancy giggled, splashing around beside me.

"Yeah, I feel like one of those lizards," Vicki added as she stretched out on a warm, flat rock. "It's just so nice to be able to lie like this, with no clothes on, and not feel self-conscious about my body, my missing breast. It's nice to be with people who understand."

We all assented and compared scars.

A serene half hour passed before we spotted our gear, bouncing on the backs of the mules, rounding the corner into camp. Reluctantly, we dressed and headed up to greet them. We hated to leave our little retreat and the special, quiet communion we had shared.

We helped unload the packs, carrying them by the handles, a climber on either end. The campsite was a broad flat area butted up against the cliffs. Boulders that had rolled down from above centuries before provided rooms for our tents and sleeping bags. For many of us, it was far too beautiful to be confined inside. We rolled out our mats and bags on the open ground, seeking shelter from the wind behind our rock walls.

"We have to get the flags up," I pointed out as soon as our personal gear was arranged. We lovingly tied strings of prayer flags together and stretched them from tent to tent, framing our camp. It was beautiful but sad, for we couldn't help but think about all the lives, some so very familiar, that had been cut short by this insidious disease.

That night after a big bowl of pasta and a mug of hot chocolate, I cozied into my sleeping bag. I tried to identify the constellations that glittered above, twinkling with hundreds of stars. But my muscles relaxed and my eyelids grew heavy, and I was lulled to sleep by the sound of the river and the flags flapping in the breeze.

We awoke in anticipation of our first water crossing. Although one doesn't think of rivers as being a treacherous part of mountain climbing, on the approach to Aconcagua they are a serious obstacle. Although we had found some still water in which to bathe, we had looked beyond the rocks that sheltered us to a river traveling with such force that anything dropped in its wake would immediately be swept downstream and lost forever.

"How do you think we are going to get across that?" Annette had asked while we stowed away our belongings.

"I'm not sure," I responded. "But it looks pretty exciting."

By 9:00 A.M., we were on the backs of our, fortunately, sure-footed mules. We gained a new appreciation for these animals as they easily ferried us across the roaring river to the other side.

We traveled approximately twelve miles our second day, from 9,000 feet to 11,000 feet, paralleling the river the whole way. The wind let up, and the sun beat down mercilessly. It was easy to feel that we were out for a pleasant day hike in the Caribbean and not on approach to one of the more deadly mountains in the world.

We stopped for lunch on a broad spit of beach that had formed in a fork of the river. While the guides prepared tuna and peanut-butter-and-jelly sandwiches, we took off our boots and allowed the fine granules of sand and cool water to ease our hot and blistered feet. Although it had been fairly easy walking up to that point, we had traversed miles of rock that shifted under our legs and cut into the soles of our boots.

As we rested, we gathered pretty little pebbles in an amazing variety of colors: turquoise, mauve, russet, gold.

"I feel like I'm at Club Med," Annette commented, sifting the vivid stones through her fingers.

"Yeah, I feel like someone is going to come over any minute with a tray of piña coladas," I added. "At any rate, this won't last, so we'd better enjoy it while we can."

As if to reinforce that statement, an hour later the mountain came into view for the first time on our trek. We stood there stunned, mesmerized by its raw beauty.

"Wow!" I commented as my eyes traveled up the long gully, then up the flanks of Aconcagua in search of the summit. "Long time coming."

"Still a long way to go," Claudia said, half to herself.

Yes, we all thought, captivated not just by the magnificent sight before us but also by what it symbolized.

Our second night's camp was set up in the shadow of what we had just seen. As the winds picked up and the temperature dropped, our thoughts were quickly transported from Club Med to the reality of our undertaking. That evening we calculated how many days we had been gone and figured that the trek team had probably landed in Argentina and would soon be headed our way. As the sky darkened, we leaned against one another and listened to Peter talk.

"The last two days have just prepared us for what lies ahead. Look at it as money in the bank. It will get tougher from here on out, and it will be important to keep up good PMA—positive mental attitude."

That night I nestled in a tent next to Annette and thought about the climb. I visualized the sliver of a trail I had seen etched in the snow above base camp, marking the progress of prior climbers. And I thought about Peter's earlier comments. "Aconcagua is really an ugly mountain, a big pile of rock." But the "Sentinel of Stone," the Spanish translation of *Aconcagua*, looked beautiful, especially cloaked in all its fresh new snow. The snow would be easier footing. Packed snow was a lot more stable than loose scree and would be a lot gentler on my ankle.

That following morning, shorts and T-shirts were replaced with long pants, fleece jackets, gloves, and hats. As we continued on toward base camp, we caught sight of the Andean condors that had followed us up the valley, keeping an eye on our progress. We chose to believe that this was a blessing and a portent of good luck.

We had not traveled far before we were forced to cross the river. The water had cut a narrow, swift swath through the hillsides, allowing little room to traverse the steep cliffs. In certain areas the eroded banks left no purchase for hands or feet, forcing us to the opposite side. At the first of these, we dropped our packs and surveyed the situation.

We spotted a large boulder upstream that had lodged midway across.

"We will string a rope through here," Peter pointed. "We'll set up a guide on either side and on the rock to assist the team."

One by one we awaited our turns, jumping from the shore to the slick rock to the jagged ground beyond. Wedged behind the rock was what appeared to be another boulder.

"Oh no," Vicki reacted as she stared. "That's a mule. One of the mules didn't make it!"

It was an unhappy sight. Although this mule wasn't one of ours, we were sad anyway. We had become attached to our mules, our couriers, and the local *caballeros* who fed and tended them. They had become part of our family. We didn't even mind when the muleteers removed the Expedition Inspiration hats we had given them after only one quick photo, replacing them with their more accustomed gaucho hats.

As we proceeded higher and higher, we caught glimpses of Aconcagua's immense peak, which heightened our anticipation. We had all enjoyed the trek in, the unexpected beauty and balmy weather, but we had come to climb and we were ready. We were being drawn forward as if by fate. The breathtaking silhouette unfolding before us was where our destiny lay.

A field of wildflowers and idyllic ponds ushered us into base camp at Plaza Argentina at 13,800 feet. We cheered our own arrival, congratulating one another with hugs. The prelims were over. We were now practically as high as the summit of Mount Rainier and had arrived at the crossroads that signified the end of the trek and the beginning of the climb.

Annette and I scouted out a roughed-out platform a short twenty feet up from where the cook tent would sit.

"How's this?" Annette asked, dropping her pack. "We have a great view of the food. . . ."

Annette and I cracked up as we struggled with our tent, fighting against the increasing winds and our giddiness on having come this far. We knew the next day we would rest, then prepare for carrying our first load of gear to Camp One. It would give us time to catch up on our diaries and one another.

However, at breakfast the following morning, Peter outlined a different scenario.

"First of all, we will build a latrine. There are lots of great rocks here that we can use to construct the walls. Then we will level an area for the other big tent. I also want us to smooth out tent platforms for the trek team."

My spoonful of granola stopped halfway to my mouth, and I looked over at Annette.

"Not my idea of a rest day," she whispered, shrugging her shoulders at the same time.

Once into it, though, we had a grand time. We were determined to build the best toilet and the largest, flattest spots for the tents. We also knew that the work was helping us acclimate, putting more "money in our banks."

As we gathered up rocks, a young woman from a nearby campsite, who had traveled here from Massachusetts, stopped in to see us.

"Hi," she said.

"Hi," we responded, taking a break. In climbing, it's one big club. Everyone is anxious to hear if you have been on the upper mountain and what the weather, the terrain, were like. We especially enjoyed seeing other women. It fueled our confidence that we could make it, too.

"Did you make the summit?" we wanted to know.

"Yes, yesterday. It was tough up there, but we had a clear day. We spent half an hour on top."

We were pleased to hear that.

"But I came over here to tell you that I think what you're doing is wonderful," she continued. "I have been following your story, and I just wanted to come over and wish you luck."

We smiled in return. Even here in the remote reaches of Argentina, people were aware of what we were doing and were excited about the project.

With our compound built, we were able to take the next day off. The morning was spent washing socks, shorts, and T-shirts in the stream and giving interviews to the documentary film crew. The sun continued to bless us, but at almost 14,000 feet, it was brutal. Some people paid the price. One hour without sunscreen and you were toast. I was foolish enough to wear a visor instead of a hat and spent the following week with my scalp flaking dead skin.

In the afternoon we shared our good-luck totems. Each of us carried a little bag of charms, feathers, and notes that fellow survivors and well-wishers had given us to take on this journey, either in their honor or in ours. As each person recited the special significance of her booty, I looked at my pouch. It had arrived in an envelope a week before the trip. My dear sister Lisa had spent hours, between work and the needs of her husband and four children, to hand-stitch the soft leather and bead the tricolor bear that adorned the front. Inside were my most treasured possessions. The Saint Christopher medal and the gold boxing glove that had kept me fighting in the hospital. There was my Sun Valley sun to bring me home safely, a feather from Sally, a picture of Buster and Roger, and the prayer flags in honor of my breast cancer buddies.

We cried as we listened to one another's stories. They were tears of sadness but also tears of joy for the mere fact that we were here doing what we were doing. Mary Yeo proudly displayed her "There's no woman like a Yeowoman" shirt covered with the names of friends of friends who had breast cancer. Annette held up the drawing done by her third-grade goddaughter, explaining, "She understood everything I was going through. She got every little bit about the disease." Someone else held up a charm engraved with the letters BLITS—because life is too short. We talked about our trekkers, wishing they could have been with us to share their totems, knowing that they had to have reached

Puenta del Inca by now and would soon cover the same ground we had.

When we had finished, I went for a walk. Plaza Argentina is a plateau of rock atop a broad glacial moraine. Fingers of valleys and low-lying hills extend for an eighth of a mile in two directions. I wandered toward the river. I needed a little quiet time. It had been an emotional few hours, and I wanted to be by myself. One of the things I enjoyed most about climbing was the solitude, the prolonged stretches where the mind can vegetate, resting in the cradle of the body as it rolls along. But this climb was different. I couldn't fade into the background The cameras were always rolling, either literally or in the eyes of the team. Everyone was upbeat and positive, but I knew what tomorrow would bring. It was going to be a grind. I was anxious to get moving. Perhaps I was weary of all the talk, all the hype. It was time to load up and go, see what we were made of, see how we would withstand the challenge of climbing the highest mountain in the Western Hemisphere.

On January 29, three days after we had arrived at base camp, we organized our gear and prepared to head up to high Camp One. Before we left, Peter picked up each of our packs, mentally calculating how much they weighed. When he set mine down, he looked at me and screwed up his face. I got the message that it might be a little heavy, and I figured I would try to leave some things behind. Maybe I didn't really need all those Stoker Bars and that extra pair of socks. I was not going to ditch my slip-on sheepskin Ugg boots. They were like fleece-lined slippers. I knew they would be much welcomed after a hard day of climbing.

This was the first of four carries. In order to establish the upper camps at 16,000 and 19,000 feet, we would have to lug up all our personal and group provisions, including tents, stoves, fuel, food, and ropes. It was too much to carry in one load, so we would take up as much as we could, stash it at 16,000 feet, then return to 13,800 to spend the night. Weather permitting, we would get up the next morning, disassemble most of the camp, and ferry it up.

It is important in expedition-style climbing to "climb high and sleep low," allowing your body the maximum opportunity to acclimate to the diminished oxygen in the atmosphere. The extra days spent ferrying our gear would increase our chances of reaching the top.

The trip to 16,000 feet woke us up to the effort that would be required to reach our goal. Our backs and shoulders weren't used to the fifty- to sixty-pound loads we had strapped to them. The steeper terrain was a combination of scree and ice, making the footing precarious. And the air was thinner. After a few days at base camp, we had backed off the pressure breathing, but now it became a necessity.

I was so focused on my breathing that at 15,000 feet I stepped on a patch of loose rock that just barely concealed black ice. As I backslid downhill, I reminded myself to concentrate even harder on where I placed my feet. My downward momentum was halted when one of the guides grabbed the straps of my pack on my way past. I would definitely be more careful.

We reached Camp One without further incident, and after unloading our gear and taking a short break, we hiked back down to base camp. We all slept well that night and were up bright and early the next day to make our move.

The first few steps of the second day on the upper mountain brought back memories of the push the day before. The first hour my pack dug into my back, and I mentally reviewed the changes I would make at the first rest break. But once I fell into a tempo, any discomfort was forgotten. I also thought about each step, carefully placed, making sure it was secure before moving on, and how that symbolizes life. *If we moved this cautiously, thoughtfully, methodically through life,* I ruminated, *we wouldn't slip back, having to catch our breath before moving on.* There is an advantage to making each step, each move through life, purposeful, headed slowly, surely toward a goal.

At the moment, I was just content to arrive at our first high camp and to have two carries behind me.

Camp One was beautiful, nestled on a small plateau between ice fields and sheer rock walls. Annette and I found a delightful cubbyhole in which to set up our tent. A six-foot flat area had been carved out among the rocks. A two-foot wall on one side and a three-foot wall on the other would provide protection against the winds. At the end of the clearing was an immense boulder standing six feet high. Stuffed under it were candy wrappers and tin cans, the obvious residue of less conscientious climbers.

As we arranged our clothing and incidentals in our temporary home, we looked out the front flap of our tent.

"Pretty nice views," I commented, looking down on the route that had brought us here.

"Not too shabby," Annette agreed.

That night the wind roared, slapping the prayer flags against the tent. I was unable to get to sleep for fear my boots, which were outside, would be whisked down the mountain. Even though they were stuffed under my pack, which was secured with a good-sized rock, I was still concerned. Reluctantly, I left the comfort of my down bag to retrieve them and reminded myself not to do that again. I got up one more time to pee, making it only a few feet from our shelter. The fierce winds whirled around me, practically lifting me off the ground and sending me south to base camp. I hopped around in the squat position, trying desperately to position myself to keep urine from spraying all over my legs. Sensing someone watching, I looked up to see Peter's face peering out of the inverted V-shaped flap of his tent, apparently amused by my predicament.

In the morning we found Dr. Bud hunched by the creek that ran through camp, staring down at his pack, which was frozen solid in the still water. It apparently had slid there, along with its securing boulder, sometime during the night.

After a day of rest, the plan was to carry to Camp Two, but the weather gods deemed otherwise. We spent a couple of hours building up rock walls, which provided a bit more relief from the wind, but the gusts increased. As we huddled outside against the tents, we observed two climbers foolishly trying to go higher. We watched them being buffeted around and could only imagine their discomfort and the added energy they were expending just to stay on their feet. We were relieved when, several hours later, we saw them turn and ease their way back down. Unfortunately, they were so wasted by the time they reached us that they had no alternative but to continue on to a lower altitude. They would not have had the strength to survive a night at 16,000 feet.

With the afternoon winds came snow, and we were confined to our tents. The day became a whirling dervish of a whiteout. Opening the flap to our tent, even for a moment, brought a blast of cold flakes inside. It was snowing so hard it was a little frightening. A small team of climbers poked their heads into our tent as they headed down. They had tossed in the towel, leaving us the remainder of their food in order to lighten their loads. I didn't envy their trip back to base camp, nor did I relish being left behind and jostled around for another night or two. Annette and I holed up, playing hearts and double solitaire, reading our paperbacks and writing in our diaries. Through the goodness of our guides, we were served a hot dinner in our tents. "Room service," Annette pointed out.

That night, the sides of our tent rattled with each blast of wind, and we snuggled deeper into our bags. The winds on Aconcagua have been described as "like a freight train coming through camp." Now I understood why. I lay there trying to calculate how much weight was in our tent. Would it be enough, I wondered, to keep us from getting lifted off the ground and cartwheeling down the mountain?

Throughout the following day and evening, the winds increased in velocity. We heard through the two-way radio that fifty- to sixty-mile-an-hour winds destroyed base camp, completely shredding the largest tents. We fretted about Jeannie Morris, who had insisted on remaining at base camp. She was writing the documentary of our climb and had wanted to be able to greet the trek team as the women and men completed their hike to Plaza Argentina. We hoped that Jeannie had been able to take refuge from the high winds. We estimated that the trekkers would be somewhere between 10,000 and 12,000 feet, and we hoped that the weather was milder at the lower elevations. We tried to remain upbeat, knowing the weather would change eventually. Yet we were aware that we had allotted only a certain number of weather days. If we weren't able to make at least one carry in the next two days, we might not have a chance for the summit.

It is easy to get stir-crazy confined to a tent. We would get out and walk around, braving the wind and cold for as long as we could bear it, then we would crawl back inside. Everything was starting to smell gamey. We tried cleaning ourselves with baby-scented wipes, but they barely made a difference. We prayed that the winds would cease. I thought about the beauty in nature's many faces—fierce and docile, inviting and intimidating, always making it clear who's boss, and I hoped "she" would be sympathetic to the purpose of our mission.

That night we had our first on-mountain communication with the trek team. We huddled as tightly as we could behind the rock wall that provided a wind break for the kitchen and waited as we listened to static on the shortwave radio.

"This is the summit team calling the trek team," Peter had just said.

Seconds dragged as we squeezed in closer, watching the radio, hoping that at any moment familiar voices would jump out of it.

"This is the trek team," came Erika's voice. "Do you copy?"

"Loud and clear," Peter responded, smiling along with the rest of us.

"How are you doing?" they wanted to know.

"We're doing fine," Peter answered. "The weather has been a little rough, but we will probably try to move tomorrow even in marginal weather."

"It's like Siberia up here," I added, and I reminded them to muscle up for their final hike into base camp. "Tomorrow will be your biggest day, so keep up the good, positive mental attitude!"

They signed off in unison, yelling their support. We went to sleep with a great deal of warmth in our hearts for the wonderful women and men who were cheering us on, and we dreamed of the wonderful celebration we would have once we were reunited.

The next two days we made trips to Camp Two despite the weather. The climb from 16,000 to 19,000 is mostly direct and exposed. We were buffeted around, but we layered up, kept our heads down, and pushed forward. The only ones not with us were Andrea Gabbard and Mary Yeo. Andrea, our team journalist, suffered from bronchitis and allergies, her face swelling up to the point that she could barely see. She knew her climb was over and accepted that fact, looking forward to getting back to base camp where she might feel better. Mary tried to climb with us, moving ever so slowly out of Camp One. But the total exertion of the last week caught up with her, and eventually she, too, realized she would be going down.

I looked down from 17,000 feet to see how those behind me were doing and caught sight of Mary's lonely figure, 900 feet below, as she struggled to put one foot in front of the other. It saddened me to know she wasn't going to make it, that the summit team was now smaller by two. I had hoped, unrealistically, that we would all stand on the summit together, holding hands and raising our flags, just as we had done lower on the mountain.

Not much was said that night. Our long-awaited dream was just around the corner. The prelims were over; now all that remained was the summit. It is an incredible feeling when so much time and effort have gone into something and suddenly you're there. As I struggled with sleep, it was hard to believe that the following day this would all be over. The outcome would be established and would become a part of history. I was looking forward to what I hoped would be a victory celebration, but it was with a touch of sadness that I closed my eyes, knowing that, for better or worse, this two-year chapter of my life was coming to a close.

CHAPTER 19

The Summit

If you have built castles in the air, your work
need not be lost; that is where they should be.
Now put foundations under them.

Henry David Thoreau

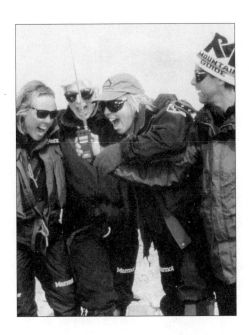

One doesn't conquer cancer or mountains. What one does conquer is the fear of death. This is important in order to truly live. I choose life, without compromise, where I will strive daily to leave fear behind and follow my instincts and dreams wherever they may take me.

———————————■———————————

I did not sleep well. I suspect nobody did. At 19,000 feet, your heart races trying to compensate for the diminished oxygen in the air. Mine was racing also for a different reason. I was still coming to terms with the fact that if the weather held this would all be over in twenty-four hours. I snuggled deeper into my sleeping bag, pulling my wool hat down over my ears. I shifted around, trying to find room for my feet among the water bottles, clothes, and energy bars that would keep me warm and fueled on the upper mountain. I was aware of the labored breathing of my two tentmates, their heads inches from mine in this small tent. I listened to the stillness of the night outside, much quieter than preceding ones, without the roar of wind we had come to expect, and I tried to calm my heart, slow my breathing, get some rest.

Roger says I climb for validation that I am well, and of course he's right. I remembered when I could barely walk, my lungs so battered by the cancer treatment. My ribs ached from the effort of constant vomiting, my body was sore from months in bed and devoid of any muscle tone I'd once had. I thought back, then rubbed the muscles in my shoulders and stretched my legs, feeling the strength in my quads and hamstrings. I had trained hard and knew that my limbs and determination would carry me up this mountain tomorrow, further away from the hospital, further away from the crippling effects of the treatment, further from the mental anguish of the disease.

I had barely shut my eyes when I could hear Peter walking around outside. A few short hours earlier, as we settled into camp, he had said, "I will check the weather around 2:00 A.M. If it's clear, we're heading up. We'll get you up at 3:30. Be ready to go. Three layers on the top, an extra layer in your pack. Make sure your ice ax, crampons, and headlamp are where you can get to them easily. It's going to be cold. You don't want to be the one to keep the rest of the team waiting."

I could vaguely hear the guides rustling around the cook tent, boiling water, digging through garbage bags for what was left of our breakfast bars. *It must be clear,* I thought. This would be the day. It took no effort to roust my tentmates, who were soon bumping elbows and heads searching for the gear that had been carefully assembled the night before.

There was nervous excitement as we quietly layered fleece over long johns, rechecking our packs for tissues, goggles, water bottles, down jackets, food. This would be a long day. *What else might I need? Will the weather hold? If not, will we miss our chance for the summit?*

Twenty-three thousand feet is a big mountain, higher than any of us had ever been. It was impossible not to wonder, *What will it be like up there? What if I don't make it?* So much was riding on this climb, highly publicized across the country, around the world. I knew I was the focal point. Everyone expected me to stand on the summit. *What if . . .*

These thoughts rattled around in our heads in the quiet of that cold, dark morning as we tediously strapped on our crampons. It had to be ten below or colder. *Will I ever warm up? Maybe, once we get moving.*

Around 5:30 A.M. we headed out. There was no full moon to guide us, only the shallow beams of light from our headlamps. I followed the line of rope in front of me, barely able to make out Peter attached to the end of it.

I could see the light in front of him bob up and down slightly, then unexpectedly drop three feet. "Oh my God!" I couldn't stop. We were roped together. Whatever had swallowed him up would be waiting for me. Just as suddenly, I found myself rib deep in snow, floundering in the icy cold of that early morning to get out of the hole that engulfed me and using up precious energy in the process.

Aconcagua is famous for its *penitentes,* spectacular spires of snow sometimes towering eight feet high, caused by the fierce winds and blowing dirt. It had snowed here nonstop for the previous three weeks, stranding all but two who had attempted the summit. The *penitentes* were now buried, the valleys in between filled with the snow we were struggling to get out of. We would pull ourselves out, take a few steps, then go down again.

After caving in two more times, no one walked any longer. We crawled, swam, rolled, and got tangled in the rope. Annette, behind me, was being pulled down the slope as the slack between us caught on my pack, around my waist.

"Laura, I need more rope," I could hear Annette panting behind me. I rolled back uphill to accommodate. I tried not to consider the fact that this was a bad way to start a long summit day, but it was difficult not to get discouraged.

We somehow reached firm ground twenty minutes later. I was relieved that firmer ground, in fact, existed. I knew we would never make it if we had to deal with rotten snow the whole way. As we caught our breath, I brushed the snow from my jacket and pants, disengaging myself from the rope coiled around me. "You okay?" Peter directed my way in the darkness. "That sucked," was my only reply.

I pushed forward. It would be another two and a half hours before we could take a break, all of us cold, exhausted, spent. The long, steep, relentless incline across the Polish Glacier would lead us to the Ruta Normal and on toward the summit. I pulled my fingers into my palms, balling up my hands inside my gloves, testing for feeling, finding little. Thankfully, I could feel my toes. For a moment I looked up from my feet at the breathtaking beauty laid out below us. Layers of mountains were tricolored in the early morning light, as the sun lifted a curtain to the day. The spectacular panorama made up for the cold.

But I could feel the rope taut behind me, could feel Annette slowing down. Kurt, in front, kept his long limbs moving forward in an attempt to warm them up, tightening the rope between us. "I need to slow down," I heard faintly from Annette.

"We have to keep moving," from Kurt.

There is a set pace in the mountains. I knew it. It is based on the amount of time it takes to get to the summit and back down safely. Annette was in trouble.

"I have to stop," came back weaker.

"Kurt, we have a problem. Annette needs to stop," I relayed.

In the seconds it took to get back to Annette, she was in a heap, on the snow, sobbing, gasping for air, her disappointment enormous. "I can't go on. I can't breathe. I let you down." I held her, reassuring her that there would be other summits, that she had not let me down, that she in fact had climbed higher than she ever had before. Besides, I reminded her, she only started climbing eight months earlier. No consolation would help, however, and I knew clearly how destroyed I would have been if it had been me instead of Annette.

It was sad to see Annette turn. I thought about her many friends, who no doubt like mine had stated, "You'll make it, you're strong." You never know. I forced myself not to think about all the people counting on me, of women in hospital rooms throughout the U.S., with pictures of the kick-ass ad tacked to their walls. "I can do 4,000 feet of vertical," I reminded myself. "Easy walking," I would say, trying to ignore the fact that I was now climbing at an altitude over 20,000 feet.

"Twenty thousand feet is where airplanes fly," Roger was fond of saying. I thought of him, at base camp, waiting patiently, confident of my abilities, anxious for me to give birth to this baby that had monopolized so much of our lives over the past two years. I thought of the rest of the team, hopeful, anticipating a successful summit, pushing us up with their support.

In my pack in a baggie were my special prayer flags. An aqua one for Susan, our dear friend from Boston, so buoyant, so full of life at one time. She was younger than I but had died in the spring, leaving behind two young boys and a grieving husband. That flag would go to the top. In her honor, in honor of all women, in honor of hope. If I didn't make the summit, hope would be diminished. "But I would, I can, I will," I recited.

I focused on one small uphill step at a time. My mantra. How many times had I repeated that in my talks, making the comparison between surviving breast cancer and climbing? I gathered energy from my rope team, from the trek team down below, and from the thousands of people supporting Expedition Inspiration. And I thought of the women in my wellness group, the flag I carried in their honor, the support we gave one another.

We climbed through three hours of darkness before we reached a level area that was safe enough to take a break. We pulled out more layers of clothing in an attempt to warm up and sat there like lumps, barely moving, for almost a half hour. When we had warmed up enough to use our hands, we pulled out the radio and informed the trek team that we were on our way. By the time we started climbing again, we had warded off the early morning chill.

Each break was welcome, a handful of M&Ms, a Stoker bar, water. Dr. Bud handing out his little white sucrose tablets. Anything for a burst of energy. Other than that, though, food didn't hold much appeal.

At 21,000 feet Vicki turned, another very sad moment. We flew our prayer flags and hugged before continuing on up. I had thought Vicki and Annette would make it, and I knew they had, too. I hoped that they wouldn't be too hard on themselves. We had now lost a total of five summit team members and were down to three breast cancer survivors: Claudia Berryman-Shafer, Nancy Knoble, and me climbing with Peter, the Doc, and the media crew. We had 2,000 feet to go.

We rested on the level ridge below the *cantaletta*, the rugged final approach to the summit of Aconcagua, bundled in our down jackets. From here on up it would get steeper. We squinted our eyes to make out two lonely climbers inching their way up the rock-littered snowfield. They looked like ants going at a snail's pace.

"After this we'll stop every twenty or thirty minutes for a short break. It will be too tough on you otherwise." I registered Peter's words as I looked up to where the summit must be, hidden behind rocks and boulders. This was going to be a difficult push. "The cantaletta is a discouraging way to finish a climb," Peter had said when we first viewed slides of Aconcagua. "If you want to go all the way, you're going to have to dig deep. You're going to have to suffer." As he spoke, I glanced at Claudia. Did Peter forget what we had been through? She had smiled. Later Peter would admit, "These team members are so much different from the average person. They've all been close to the edge, close to death. That makes them wonderful climbers. What typical people fear, they handle much better." I thought about where I'd rather be at that moment—back in the hospital isolation room or here, suffering on the side of this mountain. *Here is just fine.*

We headed up the final approach to the summit, mired down in deep snow, which was followed by loose rock and scree. I concentrated on pressure breathing, expanding my lungs to full capacity, then forcing the air out: two, three, sometimes four breaths per step. I tried to find and maintain a rhythm of sorts. Any wasted motion at that altitude would drain what vital energy was left.

The climb became more of a scramble above 22,000 feet. Large boulders forced us to take giant steps up and around them, requiring us to gasp in more air. My pin-and-screw Rainier ankle shot painful signals up my leg from repeatedly twisting it on the loose rock. And above, we could see dark clouds. Worse weather was coming in.

We were getting closer, though, pushing through the invisible barrier that tried to stop us. Fifteen feet from the summit we took our final break. Peter pulled out the shortwave radio and called down to 14,000 feet, "Base, this is the summit team. Do you copy?"

"The trek team is all here. We're looking at the mountain," came Erika's sweet voice, as if she were right beside us, not nine thousand feet below.

"We're fifteen feet from the summit," Peter continued. "We're going to make it!"

The jubilant cheers of the trek team reverberated through the radio, reducing us to tears. I could hear my husband's proud joy, "You've made all of our dreams come true." Through a mist I looked out at the resplendent beauty of nature. Stretched below us were mountains interspersed with lush valleys, including the one we had come up. A million miles away. We were going to do it. This was the first time we were clear in the knowledge that we would make the summit, that we would achieve what we had set out to achieve. The first time any of us could allow ourselves to verbalize it.

I thought of Claudia and Nancy nestled in the rock beside me. We had all suffered here on this mountain. And before. We had looked into the jaws of death, but not by choice. To take our chances there on Aconcagua, knowing the risks, made us giddy. To do something we weren't certain we could do made us stronger, opening up a world of options.

Twelve days, eleven hours, and forty minutes after we had physically begun this journey, we were truly on top of the world. We were euphoric that we had made it, grinning ear-to-ear as we took that last step onto the narrow platform that formed the summit. Three breast cancer survivors standing proudly, arm in arm, happy to be alive, more alive than ever at 23,000 feet.

I touched the prayer flags, which were now in my pocket, willing energy and hope to the millions of women who needed it. I brushed tears from my eyes for those who would not share in the glory of this moment. And I thought to myself that this was the only way I would have wanted to celebrate the five-year anniversary of my cancer diagnosis.

I also thought, for the first time, that I must be cured.

CHAPTER 20

The Descent

To be what we are and to become what we are capable of is the only end in life.

Robert L. Stevenson

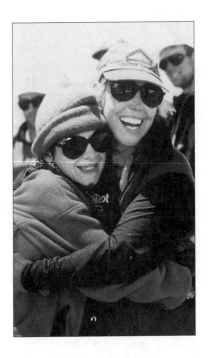

There is fear in climbing: a quiet subtle echo when you look up or down or into the yawning mouth of a crevasse. Very real danger, beckoning, reminding you clearly of the value of life. It is not fear that keeps me climbing. It is the beauty of hardship, of having endured, survived, pushed on that magnifies the beauty of everyday life.

———————■———————

What goes up must come down. But in the euphoria of having reached our goal, I temporarily lost sight of that. On the summit of Aconcagua, I let out a huge sigh of relief. We had achieved what we had set out to accomplish, at least on the mountain, and I had held up my end of the bargain. All the effort of the last two years washed away.

I looked out at the vast panorama that stretched below us, layers upon layers of peaks gradually tapering into the distance. I remembered someone having told me, "You can see the curve of the earth from the highest point in the Western Hemisphere." I strained to see beyond the mountain ranges for some indication that the world is, in fact, round, but I found none. Instead I saw, or perhaps felt, an endless expanse of hope.

I never doubted my will or determination, but I could not completely forget how traumatized my body had been from all the drugs. My oncologist later expressed her deep concern about my final approach to the summit. As she said, "As far as I know, no one who has been through the severe treatment you went through has ever climbed to these altitudes. I didn't know what to expect, how your heart and lungs would respond."

One article said what we were attempting was a miracle, but the miracle wasn't the climb. Achieving the summit demonstrated the miraculous nature of the human mind and body. It was also a demonstration of desire and the determination to go after what one wishes for. Alejandro Randis wrote in his book on Aconcagua,

> The most desired dreams, always, always become reality. And when that happens, its magic destroys the barriers of the "it can not be" and suddenly erases the limits of time. Only dreams and their magic give life its mysteries and inextinguishable bright. (From Aconcagua, El Centinele de Piedra, available only in Argentina. The book's translations are rough, much like the mountain.)

If I had been paying more attention to the fact that I now had to come off one of the highest mountains in the world and less attention to our remarkable achievement, I would not have almost killed myself on our descent.

I had taken perhaps three steps when the knifelike points of my crampons on my right foot hooked the straps that attached the same protection to my other foot. Thrown off balance, I rolled head over heels down the dreaded and treacherous *cantaletta*. I sat there stunned, aware, once again, how quickly things can change, particularly if you're not paying attention.

I assessed the damage. Luckily I had sustained only minor cuts and bruises. I was reprimanding myself when I heard Peter's firm voice, "Laura, you're okay. You had an emotional meltdown. Pull yourself together. We have a long way to go still."

As I knew. Our success would be meaningless if someone got seriously injured at this point. We had to all get down, without major mishap. I put aside all thoughts of Expedition Inspiration and what it stood for and instead concentrated on each step, summoning up every last ounce of energy I had. It was around 4:30 in the afternoon when we left the summit. Because bad weather was coming in and it was beginning to get dark, we had spent barely half an hour on top. Now it was imperative to descend as briskly as possible, to get back to high camp in what remained of the daylight and the deteriorating weather.

By the time we completed the traverse and were faced with the final uphill that led back to our tents at 19,000 feet, we had been moving for fourteen hours (eleven up and three down). Everyone was wasted. I recall our team doctor later estimating that we had burned close to fifteen thousand calories that day, about a thousand an hour. No wonder we were beat!

We dragged into camp just as the last of the light faded. After brief congratulatory hugs with the few climbers from our team and other teams who were preparing to go up or down, we headed straight for our tents. I remember vaguely trying to squeeze into the front opening of my tent with my pack on, not wishing to exert any more effort, only wanting to lie down. It didn't work, of course. So I removed my pack, crampons, and boots, ate hastily prepared lasagna, and was settled in within half an hour. I then slept, probably without even rolling over, for a solid twelve hours.

There are few things quite as invigorating as a high mountain morning. The air is so fresh, tinged with a light chill that helps to get the mind and muscles moving. The view is no less than spectacular, as the early morning sun blankets the hillsides with a collage of color. The steaming cup of hot chocolate or coffee tastes better than a five-star meal. But that particular high altitude morning was also filled with the excitement of what lay below—our team. We were anxious to share the joy of our victory, to see our comrades, many of whom we hadn't seen for months, not since the last team meeting in Sun Valley. Because the Expedition Inspiration team members resided throughout the United States, from Washington State to Maine, we had had only two get-togethers. One had been the shakedown climb on Mount Rainier, the other a media event and fund-raiser in Idaho.

Rested and refreshed, we leisurely broke camp, packed up, and started down. We could make out a few familiar faces as we trekked into Camp One at 16,000 feet, but the majority of the support team members were still on their way up from base camp. I could barely contain myself. I couldn't wait to see my husband's proud face and the faces of my fellow survivors and friends who over the last year had become like family.

I ran down to greet them as they appeared over the rocky rise below camp. I hugged my husband first, enjoying a big sloppy kiss, then embraced each of our wonderful support team members. Everyone was ecstatic that the climb had been a success and that we had returned safely.

Last was my oncologist, Dr. Kathleen Grant. I felt in a very big way that I owed this success to her. If it hadn't been for her soft-spoken encouragement, I would not have entered into the bone marrow trial that I was certain had saved my life.

I thought about the many doctors and nurses who had said, "We don't hear about the survivors." And I thought about how pleased Dr. Grant must be to see one of her patients not only survive but achieve what many thought impossible. I had to tell her how I felt.

As I squeezed my arms around her, I said, "Kathleen, you're the reason I'm here."

She quickly replied, "No, no, you're the reason I'm here."

By the time we reached base camp, a celebration was clearly in order, but we were unprepared for the surprise that awaited us, compliments of the support team and our guides. In a large cooler by the cook tent were twenty bottles of champagne and two scrumptious looking cheesecakes.

After solar showers and what would suffice for clean clothes, we partied. Word of our successful summit and our mission had spread throughout the Plaza Argentina's base camp, and we were soon joined by well-wishers from all parts of the world. Fortunately, there were many people to help with the champagne, since alcohol at high altitude, in this case 13,800 feet, can have dizzying effects. I'm sure there were a few onlookers who were convinced this was the case when Annette Porter and Eleanor Davis, as a surprise for the team, crept out of a tent in minidresses, fishnet hose, high heels, and neon Tina Turner wigs. Posed as Tess and Terry, twins, they gyrated to "What's Love Got to Do with It" for as long as their lungs held out.

We laughed till we cried, and we rejoiced in the beauty of life.

CHAPTER 21

Down from the Mountain

A life has to move or it stagnates. . . . I have had
responsibilities and work, dangers and pleasure,
good friends, and a world without walls to live in.

Beryl Markham

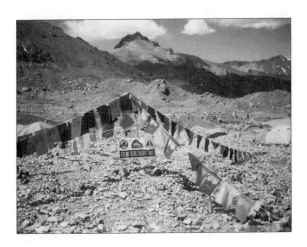

I will try to live my life by the five C philosophy: Courage, Commitment, Consistency, Confidence, and Control. Perhaps if I am able to maintain my strength and conviction, others will do the same.

———————■———————

The Aconcagua climb was one of those life experiences I hope I never forget. It will always be a memory of a special time and place, to be cherished for years to come—not just for me, but for every member on the team. We had shared a part of our souls with each other and with breast cancer survivors around the world.

All of us learned a great deal about ourselves. For me, the lessons were about leadership and the responsibility that goes with it. For many, it was the unexpected thrill of pushing the envelope, of going beyond where they had ever ventured before. For members of the team who didn't make it as far as they had hoped, it meant learning to let go. For every one of us, it meant gaining an even greater appreciation for the value of support.

On a grander scale, we knew that our efforts and the Expedition Inspiration documentary had done more than perhaps any other single project to raise awareness about the breast cancer epidemic. Through the Expedition Inspiration Fund for Breast Cancer Research and the Breast Cancer Fund, we raised close to two million dollars, which would be allocated for cutting-edge projects that will eventually lead to a cure. We had made a valuable contribution to society, for which we were all proud. But an obligation went with it, and we knew it. Each of us would continue, either with Expedition Inspiration or in our own way, to help others and to work for the breast cancer cause.

Sitting on that plane on our return trip to the United States, gazing down at the broad expanse of land below, I enjoyed a brief respite from the hard work of the climb and the project as a whole. But I recognized that my quiet time would be brief. There would be more Expedition Inspirations. I knew that as long as I was able, I would continue the positive momentum we had started.

I feel fortunate to be alive, to have achieved goals that were once only soft whispers in the night, floating through my subconscious mind. If through my continued efforts I can help others deal with breast cancer, or any crisis, and help them feel as I did the moment I stood on the top of the Western Hemisphere, then what an incredible payback. How rare it is that we discover the gift we have to give! I count myself among the very lucky.

I often smile to myself when I think of my favorite cartoon. It is an illustration of a man looking at a flyer tacked to a tree. The caption reads:

L O S T
Hunting Dog. 3 Legs. Tail broken.
Blind in one eye. Left ear missing.
Recently neutered. Answers to
name "Lucky."

The sentiment sums up exactly how I feel. Like the dog in the cartoon, I, too, had altered body parts. And like the dog, I, too, would call myself lucky. As I climb through life, I will always remember the sad-looking Lucky dog in that poster and will carry with me a great appreciation for life, in all its unpredictable forms.

I will also keep close to mind these words: "May the winds call out our courage and strength. May we find peace in remembrance. May we triumph over illness."

Laura Evans 1995

ONE STEP AT A TIME.

ONE STEP AT A TIME.

ONE STEP AT A TIME.

ONE STEP AT A TIME.

ONE STEP AT A TIME.

ONE STEP AT A TIME.

ONE STEP AT A TIME.

ONE STEP AT A TIME.

ONE STEP AT A TIME.

ONE STEP AT A TIME.

ONE STEP AT A TIME.

ONE STEP AT A TIME.

ONE STEP AT A TIME.

ONE STEP AT A TIME.

ONE STEP AT A TIME.

ONE STEP AT A TIME.

Laura Evans 1990

What is it about faith and mountains, that someone who could barely climb out of bed would eventually reach 23,000 feet? Congratulations to Laura Evans and the team of breast cancer survivors who conquered Mt. Aconcagua to fight the disease that nearly killed them.

EXPEDITION INSPIRATION

©1995 JanSport, Inc.

On May 1, 1995, the Expedition Inspiration team was honored by Hillary Rodham Clinton at a private reception in the White House. The team also met with fellow breast cancer survivor Sandra Day O'Connor and several members of Congress to help underscore the urgency for the government to allocate more research dollars to help curb the breast cancer epidemic.

On July 12, 1995, the PBS documentary film of Expedition Inspiration was aired nationally. Jeannie Morris of Bill Kurtis Productions wrote and produced the film, doing a remarkable job of capturing the essence of Expedition Inspiration. In viewing the film, women and men alike were affected by the profound determination and will of the women on the screen. One young man in his early twenties came up to me afterward and said, "I have never been sick a day in my life, but your documentary showed me that I can overcome anything I confront." Another woman commented that her husband wouldn't even talk about breast cancer, even though she was battling it, until he saw the coverage of Expedition Inspiration.

A second Expedition Inspiration climb has been scheduled for Mount Vinson, in Antarctica, in December of 1996. Remote and challenging, with extreme climatic conditions, Mount Vinson presents itself as an excellent vehicle for another team of dauntless survivors to call attention to the disease that almost took their lives.

In addition to conducting major climbs, Expedition Inspiration will be telling breast cancer to "Take-a-Hike" by conducting locally organized and sponsored hike-a-thons under this name across all of North America. The hiking events were begun to include the hundreds of people who have expressed an interest in being involved with Expedition Inspiration's message to raise awareness, funds, and hope. The first successful hike took place in Seattle in October of 1995.

In 1996 Canada joined in the mission and objectives of Expedition Inspiration by recruiting climbers and sponsors for both the international expeditions and local hikes. It is our hope that in the not-too-distant future, Expedition Inspiration will have team members from countries throughout the world. We will be the visible survivors, but many more will be with us in spirit.

The numbers of women contracting breast cancer are staggering. In 1995 it was reported in the *Journal of the American Medical Association,* "In the past two decades, breast cancer has claimed more lives than the total fatalities of the Korean War, the Vietnam War, World War I and World War II combined."

What is more frightening, we don't know why. Through the combined efforts of a talented board of directors and outstanding medical board, the Expedition Inspiration Fund for Breast Cancer Research will educate women and men in advances made in diagnosing, treating, and assisting in the recovery from breast cancer. The fund will work closely with renowned doctors, researchers, and research hospitals in the breast cancer field to determine which projects will have the greatest impact in alleviating the effects of and finding a cure for breast cancer.

Part of the proceeds from this book will be donated to:

The Expedition Inspiration Fund for Breast Cancer Research

To find out how you can help or to make a donation, write to:

P.O. Box 4289
Ketchum, Idaho 83340

Phone: 208.726.6456
Fax: 208.726.2040

Recommended reading:

You Cannot Afford the Luxury of a Negative Thought, by John-
    Roger and Peter McWilliams
Lou Whittaker, by Andrea Gabbard
Touching the Void, by Joe Simpson
West with the Night, by Beryl Markham
Talk Before Sleep, by Elizabeth Berg
Picasso's Woman, by Rosalind MacPhee

To learn more about mountaineering, contact:

Summits Adventure Travel
51902 Wanda Road
Eatonville, Washington 98328
Phone: 360.569.2992
Fax: 360.569.2993